THE
LIFE
PLAN
DIET

Also by Jeffry S. Life, MD, PhD

Mastering the Life Plan

The Life Plan

THE LIFE PLAN DIET

How Losing Belly Fat Is the Key to Gaining a Stronger, Sexier, Healthier Body

Jeffry S. Life, MD, PhD

ATRIA BOOKS

New York   London   Toronto   Sydney   New Delhi

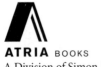

ATRIA BOOKS
A Division of Simon & Schuster, Inc.
1230 Avenue of the Americas
New York, NY 10020

This publication contains the opinions and ideas of its author. It is intended to provide helpful and informative material on the subjects addressed in the publication. It is sold with the understanding that the author and publisher are not engaged in rendering medical, health, or any other kind of personal or professional services in the book. The reader should consult his or her medical, health, or other competent professional before adopting any of the suggestions in this book or drawing inferences from it.

The author and publisher specifically disclaim all responsibility for any liability, loss, or risk, personal or otherwise, which is incurred as a consequence, directly or indirectly, of the use and applications of any of the contents of this book.

First Atria Books hardcover edition March 2014

ATRIA BOOKS and colophon are trademarks of Simon & Schuster, Inc.

For information about special discounts for bulk purchases, please contact Simon & Schuster Special Sales at 1-866-506-1949 or business@simonandschuster.com.

The Simon & Schuster Speakers Bureau can bring authors to your live event. For more information or to book an event, contact the Simon & Schuster Speakers Bureau at 1-866-248-3049 or visit our website at www.simonspeakers.com.

Jacket design by Alan Dingman
Jacket art by Jason Ellis Photography

Manufactured in the United States of America

10   9   8   7   6   5   4   3   2   1

Photographs on page 121 by Thomas F. George;
all other photographs by Jason Ellis Photography

ISBN 978-1-4767-4356-1
ISBN 978-1-4767-4358-5 (ebook)

To my wife, Annie, who was the first to motivate me to start this journey, and believed that I could win the Body-for-LIFE contest in 1998. She has supported me and my mission ever since.

Contents

THE
LIFE
PLAN
DIET

Introduction

By all accounts, I'm an incredibly lucky man. At 75 years old I'm in better health and in better physical shape compared to any other point of my life, and frankly, to most men my age and younger. I lead a vibrant, exciting life that includes travel and spending lots of time with my family, as well as continually challenging myself professionally and personally. While other men my age are set in their retirement, I can't stop thinking about the future: what else is in store for me and how I can continue to effect change. There is no secret that everyone, and everything, is going to age. My important message that I want to get out to men is that we don't have to get old as we age.

I'm also keenly aware that the last 16 years have been a gift, because if you knew me back then, you would have thought that by now I wouldn't even be here to write this book. And that's why my story is so important for every man to hear, because *I was you*. I know how to change the way you age because I have done it and am continuing to do the work today.

In early 1998, I was 59 years old, and I was honestly ready to throw in the towel. I had reached an all-time low in terms of my self-esteem, mood, level of fitness, and appearance. I had spent my entire career as a family medical practitioner in private practice in West Virginia and Pennsylvania. Even though my business was thriving, I had really lost enthusiasm for my work. Worse, I looked and felt like an old man. My joints and muscles ached, I had shortness of breath whenever I climbed just one flight of stairs, my clothes were tight, and my stomach was huge. My LDL (bad cholesterol) scores were sky high, my HDL (good cholesterol) numbers were rock bottom, I was well on my way to becoming a full-blown type 2 diabetic, and I had just learned that I had advanced heart disease. On top of all this, my interest in sex was almost nonexistent. I suffered from erectile dysfunction, and I fought a daily battle with anxiety and depression.

The irony, of course, was that I was a physician certified in family medicine who should have known about staying fit and eating right. But that's exactly what the issue was: I didn't know. Like most in my profession, I had no nutritional or exercise training, and I knew nothing about the importance of hormone therapies and their relationship to healthy aging. As a result, I had become just another middle-aged doctor who was trained to disconnect the image in the mirror from the fact that my overall health was in massive decline.

Then, one day, I found a copy of *Muscle Media* magazine lying in my exam room. I took it home that night and read it cover to cover. I couldn't believe how physically fit these men and women were, and for the first time in my life, I was jealous enough to do something about the way I looked. I signed up that night for a lifetime subscription. Soon after, I started working with my first personal trainer, Ernie Baul. When I walked into his gym I was met by a 50-year-old former Navy SEAL who took one look at me and said, "I don't know, old man. You look like quite a challenge." That was exactly what I needed to hear: His challenge would become my challenge.

One month into his balls-to-the-wall program I read about the first winners of the 1997 Body-*for*-LIFE contest. I looked at the before-and-after pictures of the participants and thought to myself, *These people can't be for real.* I was amazed at the way so many people were able to transform themselves in such a short period of time, from being fat and out of shape to being fit and lean. I showed it to Annie, my girlfriend (and now my wife), and she said, "If those contestants could transform their bodies so can you. You need to do this, Jeff . . . start now!" I didn't realize it at the time, but what she said would become the pivotal moment that has truly saved my life.

I raced to have my "before" pictures taken, then I told Ernie what I wanted to do. I had just 19 weeks to make a significant change in every aspect of my life. I gave up all of my old habits—including drinking and eating way too much—and put myself on a low-glycemic/low-fat diet that I've been following ever since, and that diet is what forms the basis of the program outlined in this book. I started taking supplements and plunged into an exercise program that I was really not prepared for. Quite honestly, the first few weeks were pretty rough: I felt exhausted, sore, and beat up most of the time. Five mornings a week I would get up at 4:00 a.m. and drive to Ernie's gym. I had to train very early in the morning so I could get my hospital rounds in and make it to my office by 9:00 a.m. Ernie taught me how to lift weights, how to build muscle and strength, how to eat clean, and how to lose body fat. He showed me how taking small steps consistently can turn into huge strides. Most important, he helped me reach down deep inside myself and maximize every last bit of my potential. He gave me the desire to set goals as high as possible and gave me the tools to reach those goals in small, yet precise, steps. He taught me the importance of working outside my comfort zone in order to achieve the changes I needed.

Nineteen weeks is not a long time to make a complete transformation, and there were many, many days when I thought I just wasn't going to be able to make it. Yet gradually I began to see real results. My LDL (bad cholesterol) went from 164 down to 80, and I started feeling better and stronger. But the mirror told the story: I could see significant changes in my physique every time I took out my "before" photos and compared them to the new me. I was beginning to like the way I looked for the first time since I graduated from medical school in 1975.

I also became obsessed with the connection between what I ate and how I felt. I read everything I could about improving nutrition, and I began a master's degree program in sports nutrition and exercise science at Marywood University in Scranton, Pennsylvania. I was taking classes with a highly motivated group of 20-year-olds while continuing to practice family medicine full-time and preparing for the Body-*for*-LIFE challenge. Yet for the first time in years I had all the energy I needed to make it through those grueling months. Looking back, I loved every one of those days.

By the end of 1998 I was just about to turn 60, and I had completed the Body-*for*-LIFE competition. I'd submitted my "before" and "after" pictures four months earlier. A few weeks before my birthday, Bill Phillips's mother called and told me I was one of the finalists in my age category. Then, on Monday, December 7, I got a call from Porter Freeman, the 1997 winner in my age category, who was then and continues to be my role model. Porter immediately asked, "What would you do, Dr. Life, if you were the winner?" I thought he was just jerking me around until he told me the real news: I *was* the winner. In just 19 weeks I went from being a dumpy old man to becoming a Grand Champion body builder who had just won a brand-new Corvette and $10,000 and transformed not only my physique but also my health.

I immediately started incorporating the program that I followed into my medical practice, trying to get every man who came into my office to experience what I had just gone through. Before my transformation I was practicing medicine the way I had been taught: providing care that was centered on treating existing disease. But once I realized how much better I felt by taking a proactive approach, I began to change my focus to disease prevention, and I attempted to get my patients to start improving their health through better eating and exercise. It was tough going at first because many of my patients were just like most American men: They thought that their chance of looking and feeling better as they got older was just about zero. But as they heard my story and saw my results, many of them started to come on board. I always started with cleaning up their diet, and then once they were beginning to see results I would get them on an exercise program based on their current health status. I stand by this approach, which is why it is perfectly fine for you to start my program by changing your diet.

I continued to train consistently and ate pretty clean, but four years later, I began to notice that I was losing ground—gaining abdominal fat and losing muscle mass as well as strength, plus my energy and sexual function were beginning to decline again. It was frustrating, to say the least, because my regimen hadn't changed: I was training as hard as ever but not seeing the same results. Everything was becoming more difficult, whether it was getting up and practicing medicine, going to the gym, or making love with my wife.

Then, in 2003, I met several Cenegenics Medical Institute doctors, as well as Dr. Alan Mintz and John Adams, the founders of this nationally known medical practice. I learned then that they promoted an exercise and nutrition program in combination with correcting hormonal deficiencies, which at the time was completely unconventional, cutting-edge medicine. I was intrigued, and I joined the Cenegenics physician training program in age-management medicine. At the same time I decided to get my own levels checked, and I learned I had major deficiencies in testosterone, DHEA, and growth hormone. That explained why I was losing muscle mass, strength, and endurance—and why I also was accumulating belly fat and battling low energy levels, sluggish thinking, and even depression. The diminished hormones also explained the other major wall I had hit: a decrease in sexual function.

I became a patient of Cenegenics in June 2003. Within two months I had already noticed profound changes in my physique and energy levels. My physician had corrected my hormone deficiencies while I continued my low-glycemic/low-fat nutrition program, combined with the right exercise and key supplements. I went from exhausted to exhilarated once again, and I also started losing belly fat and gaining clarity in my thinking, not to mention that my sexual function had improved. In January of 2004 I became a senior institute physician for Cenegenics and moved out to Las Vegas, and I've been here ever since. In 2006, Cenegenics began using my image for their marketing campaign, which they continue to do to this day (but with a more recent photo, of course).

In 2007 I ran into another roadblock. I was almost 10 years into maintaining a healthy lifestyle and excellent physical shape, yet my cardiologist was still concerned about my heart. Even though I was doing everything right, the advanced heart disease caused by my poor habits from the first 60 years of my life required that I get two stents. I was devastated, but then I realized that if I had never started taking care of myself I would not be alive at all. What's more, it's made me even more determined to prevent heart disease from happening to anyone else: This has become my mission in life.

And the rest, as they say, is history. It has now been 16 years since I began my complete physical transformation. I've been fortunate enough to be able to share my story with thousands of men all over the world so that they can achieve what I have: an enhanced level of fitness and great health. Best of all, not only do I feel great, but I've been able to improve my physique and my good health over all these years. In fact, in many ways, I'm stronger, healthier, and more fit than I was when I first got into shape. I've been able to stay strong and lean, reduce my cholesterol levels, reduce chronic or "silent" inflammation, reduce blood sugar levels, eliminate biomarkers for heart attack and stroke, and avoid diabetes. My exercise stress tests have continued to improve year after year.

Every day I'm grateful that I've been able to sustain this good health. And I'm absolutely amazed that at 75 years old, I have six-pack abs. Even though I exercise every single day, I'm still shocked when I look at myself in the mirror. I never would have believed that a 75-year-old man could have this body. I sure didn't believe it before I started. Now I believe it, because I achieved it. I look at all the guys I know in their 40s, 50s, 60s, and 70s who have huge bellies. I'm sure these men think that there is no way in the world they could ever, ever, have a six-pack. But I'm here to tell you that you can, and that's what this book is all about.

Other people I meet are just as astounded by the fact that I have a six-pack as I am. Once, when I was lecturing in Brazil, I was interviewed for a radio show and the host asked me if I had abdominal implants. I never even heard of that! But it just goes to show you how many people find it unfathomable that a guy my age can be in such good shape.

Having six-pack abs is not only my badge of fitness; it is also how I outwardly show the full extent of my internal health. In order to achieve a six-pack, you have to get rid of visceral fat, which is considered by most experts to be the single best predictor of heart disease. If you can have six-pack abs, then you have really reduced your risk for having a heart attack or stroke. Studies have shown that young men with weak abdominal muscles are at the greatest risk for dying early, before age 55. And if you're older, the impact your gut has on the rest of your health is profound, to say the least.

Now It's Your Turn

Whether you are 26 or 80 or anywhere in between, it's not too late to get with my program, which can literally change your life. And just as I did, we're going to start off by cleaning up your diet. The reason is simple: You can exercise 24 hours a day, but you won't get as much out of any of that time unless you are eating properly. My strategies for weight loss will help you evolve from a sedentary lifestyle to an active one, but you need to start by eating right in order to fully support your exercise program.

Your first goal is to commit to the progressive Life Plan Diet for at least eight weeks, and then switch over to my first book, *The Life Plan*, and start adding vigorous exercise to your daily routine. Once you start noticing the changes that accompany weight loss—to your body, your thinking, and your energy levels—you'll be even more motivated to get to the gym. Besides building strength and muscle, a cardio workout will further speed up your body fat loss, and weight lifting will help you burn more calories all day long.

Having a six-pack means that I have a strong abdomen. However, you should know that even though I eat clean and exercise every day, I spend under 30 minutes a week working my abs. Sit-ups and crunches are not what gets you a six-pack: It simply comes from reducing body fat. That's why I'm convinced that you don't need rigorous exercise to get you on track to significant fat loss, especially if you are very out of shape. I want you to start dropping body fat immediately, because that will ultimately put you in a better position to successfully exercise—both physically and psychologically. You'll be more likely to achieve your goals when you aren't overwhelmed and can focus on just one part of the program at a time. Then, when you start to drop body fat and start to get in better shape, you can ease into a formalized exercise program and experience ever better results.

You should also know that this diet isn't exactly exercise-free. You will be doing moderate walking right from the beginning. You'll begin to build up your cardiovascular endurance slowly. This is especially important for men with a lot of belly fat. The little bit of walking will also keep your mind off your old, bad eating and drinking habits, and reinforce making better food choices as you follow the diet.

The truth is that foods we choose to eat profoundly affect our physical and mental health, our athletic performance, and how we age. Researchers are continuing to uncover the direct links between poor food choices and the frightening increase in chronic diseases such as diabetes, heart disease, obesity, and Alzheimer's disease. Yet even though I know exactly which foods will make me sick, and certainly make me look and feel older, it is often not enough to stop me from eating things I know are bad for me. It is a constant, daily battle for me and my patients; a battle that I have learned how to win, and one that you can win as well.

I'm not going to lie to you: The challenging exercise program that I put myself on 16 years ago has been easy to keep up with when compared to my continuing war with what I want to put into my mouth. My relationship with food and drink has always been the toughest aspect of my own personal health journey. Before my transformation, I ate too many of the wrong foods, and way too much of them—breads, white rice, ice cream, any and all chocolates, all kinds of sweets, breakfast cereals, fried foods; the list goes on and on. Like most men, I'm still battling with a borderline consumption disorder, and it doesn't end with food. I'm the first to admit that I can easily drink way too much. Even today, if I start eating the wrong foods or drinking alcohol it isn't long before I'm completely off track.

I also know that my experience with eating is similar to that of most of my patients. It's hard work to really eat clean and exercise properly, especially in the United States. There are so many easily accessible food and drink temptations, it's no wonder so many dieters fail. Most of us live in areas where we drive around all the time instead of walk, which is another reason why so many men almost unknowingly let their health go. Then, when they're totally out of shape, it's very difficult to start a program and make a significant difference. Yet I know firsthand that it can be done. If you can win the eating battle, you can win the war against excess body fat and poor health. By avoiding the foods and beverages that can make you sick as well as fat and can ultimately kill you, you'll see a complete reversal in the signs and symptoms of aging, and you will drop those unnecessary, unhealthy pounds and increase your metabolism and energy levels.

The first step is to understand why you need to lose weight in the first place. Part One of this book will show you exactly how your weight—and specifically your belly fat—is affecting your physical, mental, and sexual health: three areas that men surely cannot let go. You'll learn how to determine how much fat you really need to lose and how much muscle you need to gain, and create a strategy based on your current health for moving forward so that you can assess all of the real, positive changes you'll achieve.

Part Two then shows exactly how to shed those pounds. You'll learn how to choose the best foods that can improve your health and help you achieve your fat-loss goals efficiently. There are four distinct diets that work together: You'll move effortlessly through them, or choose the one that works best for you in terms of your current health, your existing exercise program, and your goals. The first is a JumpStart program, which is an excellent way to drop weight quickly, especially if you haven't dieted or exercised before. This new plan has gotten rave reviews from my patients, who have lost an average of 15 pounds in just two weeks. Most important, it's a total mind-reset diet that will transition you from bad habits to good ones in just a few days.

The remaining three diets have each been featured in my two previous books, *The Life Plan* and *Mastering the Life Plan*. In this edition, I've included more of Annie's meal plans, recipes, and food options for you to work with while you follow the Basic Health, the Fat-Burning, or the Heart Health Diet. You'll choose one of these diets to follow once you've completed the JumpStart Diet, and you can stay with any of these diets forever, or move up the ladder to a more restrictive diet when you reach a plateau or are ready for a new challenge. You'll move along at your own pace while enjoying foods I know that you're going to love. Once you're on the right track, you can add the rigorous exercise programs I've outlined in my other books for the best results.

Part Three adds the missing piece that almost all other diet books fail to include: how to achieve and maintain weight loss success as you get older. Women already know that it gets harder each year to lose weight and get into shape, but the truth is, it's just as difficult for men. The reason is an insidious drop in hormone levels. For men, correcting hormone deficiencies through either food, exercise, or medical therapies may be the final piece needed for you to lose weight faster than ever, and keep it off. Addressing declining hormone levels is safe and effective, and not doing so just may be what's holding you back from achieving success.

I'm thrilled that you've chosen to begin this journey with me. I know that if you stick with this program you simply can't fail. The only thing you'll lose is the burden of the weight you've been carrying.

PART ONE

LOSE WEIGHT AND GET MORE OUT OF LIFE

CHAPTER 1

Age Management through Waist Management

The one area of the body that disappoints most men, especially as they get older, is their stomach. Abdominal or visceral obesity—what we often refer to as the pot belly or beer gut—is such a common occurrence that most men think of their expanding waistline as a rite of passage or a normal part of aging that can't be changed. This is, in fact, partially true: As men get older, they are at much greater risk for developing belly fat. But let me tell you, adjusting your belt a notch every few years is not "normal," and it's the one part of your body that can eventually do you more harm than good. That's why this book focuses almost exclusively on lightening the load that's resting at your belly.

Belly fat results from an excess production of body fat that is deposited inside the abdominal cavity, packed between and around your internal organs. This is referred to as visceral fat and is composed of several types of fat deposits, including mesenteric, epididymal white adipose tissue, and perirenal fat: This combination is one of the reasons why it is so difficult to get rid of it. Another reason is human evolution. The male belly evolved to be the great repository for stored fat, which was burned as needed in order to keep our distant cavemen ancestors alive through periods of famine. Fortunately for most of us, famine is no longer an issue, yet our bodies are still programmed to desperately hold on to excess fat stores at the waist for a future need that practically never arises.

There are many factors that may cause an increase in the production of belly fat, which range from what some would consider the most obvious to what others find highly speculative. We do know that when a person takes in more calories from food than his or her body can expend, the excess is converted into body fat and stored for later use. When we continue this cycle on a daily basis the stored fat is never required, and therefore accumulates all over the body: in the arms, legs, and most noticeably, the belly. Yet we don't know exactly why some men store more excess weight than others. The widespread misperception is that it is simply the result of eating too much or exercising too little. While maintaining a proper diet and exercising regularly do matter, these environmental influences alone cannot always determine an individual's waistline. For example, many men who are overly fat eat a relatively clean diet, exercise daily, and still have trouble losing weight.

Some studies will point out that body fat may be related to the excessive consumption of one nutrient group over another, relating weight gain to eating too much fat or carbohydrates, or foods with gluten. This is why fad diets exist. Those are the ones that are based on a study or two that suggest you forgo one particular food group in order to lose weight. Yet the next year another study shows something entirely different. These fad diets are often hard to maintain because the results are often only temporary: When you entirely forgo a particular nutrient group you may achieve real weight loss, but then other physical or emotional stresses can arise that the body has to respond to, and instead of focusing on burning body fat your body simply gets used to your new way of eating. More often than not, after the end of a couple of weeks you're back to where you started in terms of your weight. Or worse, the body has overcompensated, leading to more cravings and weight gain. And all along the way you've lost the positive aspects those nutrients hold that the rest of your body needs to function optimally.

There has been real scientific evidence that the foods we eat can affect how we look and feel. Science is pretty much in agreement that highly processed foods are one of the major culprits of the obesity epidemic here in the United States. Americans have a real dependence on readily available, highly processed food that our bodies rapidly assimilate into sugar and then mainline right into our bloodstreams, leading to insulin resistance and type 2 diabetes. However, there are also foods that can make a real positive impact on our health and our waistline. For example, we now know that the quality of protein one eats is inversely related to one's percent of abdominal fat. Quality protein is defined as having a high ratio of essential amino acids within each type of dietary protein. In other words, the less quality protein or the fewer essential amino acids we consume, the more at risk we are for developing abdominal fat. Essential amino acids are found in lean red meats, chicken, fish, protein shakes, some dairy products, such as cottage cheese and yogurt, beans, legumes, and egg whites. While you are following the Life Plan Diet, you will be having a quality protein in each and every meal, along with the proper amounts of the right dietary fats and complex carbohydrates. This perfect balance ensures that not only will you lose weight, you'll also be getting a full complement of all the nutrients your body and brain require, and you'll feel full and satisfied throughout the day.

Other research points to abdominal weight gain as genetically predetermined: If your parents were overweight you might have a gene that predisposes you to the same fate. Others blame the environment: not the air we breathe, but the environment we create, or that has been created around us. Studies show that when you hang around with people who are overweight, you will gain weight as well. A 2007 *New York Times* article reported that studies of both animal and human populations put weight gain firmly in the hands of one's mother and her lifestyle choices during pregnancy. According to the article, it's surprising but true that mothers who ate sparingly during their pregnancy were likely to have children who grew into fat adults. Other studies point out that children are more likely to be fat if their mothers smoked during pregnancy. While all of these things may be true, it's clearly too late to continue to blame your mother or your friends for your expanding waistline. You need to start taking responsibility for your own health, because it's your future that you must protect.

Our stressful lifestyle is another culprit. Elevated levels of the stress hormone cortisol are thought to contribute to abdominal obesity. Cortisol is the hormone released by the adrenal glands in response to crisis. One of the most pronounced aspects of a high-cortisol state is a shutdown of digestive activity. During periods of stress, the brain instructs the body to prioritize its functions, and one of the first to go is the proper digestion of food. The body shifts its energy away from digestive functions and toward the extremities, making them ready for fighting or fleeing. If there was a real emergency, you would be glad that your body has this built-in intelligence. But this reflex works against you when stress is part of your daily existence, be it your work life, your home life, or even the way you are constantly worrying about your weight.

A secondary effect of cortisol is that it increases the production of insulin, the fat-storing hormone. Insulin is your body's most effective way of preserving calories gained from digestion and storing them for later use. Unfortunately, these calories are converted into body fat, and when there is excess cortisol production, this fat typically accumulates around and inside the abdomen. The cortisol/insulin response was created thousands of years ago when a common trigger of stress was famine or lack of food: The body responded by slowing metabolism and storing belly fat in order to tap into vital nutrients for later use. However, each time we stress about something, the brain recognizes the shift and will release more insulin, and your body will reflexively store calories instead of burning them.

As Your Waistline Grows, Your Health Plummets

Aside from the way excess belly fat makes you look, it is affecting the way you feel right now. Your weight affects every aspect of how your body functions. Carrying around more than 10 pounds of body fat can make you experience any or all of the following:

- Anxiety

- Back pain

- Cravings for carbs (French fries, pizza, beer) or high-sugar foods (fruit, ice cream, cookies)

- Cravings for food even when you know you're not hungry

- Depression

- Diminished sexual function

- Fatigue

- Feeling old

- Fluid retention and swollen legs

- Increased difficulty exercising

- Loss of stamina

- Low self-esteem

- Poor posture

- Shortness of breath

- Sleep issues

- Slow moving

- Sore joints

- Sore muscles

Your long-term health outlook isn't all that great either if you are carrying around a spare tire. In 2013, the American Medical Association officially recognized obesity as a disease, and one that is linked to an increase in your risk for developing other serious conditions, including heart disease, type 2 diabetes, high blood pressure, stroke, liver disease, sleep apnea, osteoarthritis, and Alzheimer's disease. Scientists have also come to recognize that body fat, instead of body weight, is the key to evaluating obesity and the adverse consequences to your health. In a 2013 article published in the *Journal of the American College of Cardiology*, researchers found that excess stomach fat is significantly more dangerous than fat located in other places on the body over the long term. The study revealed that people with excessive abdominal fat have greater risk of heart disease and cancer than those with a similar weight who carry fat in other areas of the body. In fact, there is no better indicator of premature death than a large belly. If you want to live a long and healthy life, abdominal weight gain is the number-one thing you've got to avoid. More important, it's never too late to get rid of the extra pounds you are currently carrying in your belly.

Belly Fat Is the Worst Kind of Body Fat

Belly fat doesn't just hang out quietly, like the fat on your arms and legs or under your skin (subcutaneous fat), or intramuscular fat, which is found within the muscle fibers. The belly is an especially dangerous place for fat to build up, because it is located close to vital organs and their blood supply. Abdominal fat can collect inside these organs, making them less efficient. And as it increases, your belly fat literally takes on a life of its own, and it begins operating as a separate organ that produces and releases free fatty acids and dangerous inflammatory hormones that affect your entire body, causing accelerated aging, heart disease, stroke, type 2 diabetes, cancer, and Alzheimer's disease. And the bigger your belly gets, the more it secretes these harmful by-products.

The first type of secretions is a group of inflammatory hormones called *adipokines*. Because these molecules alter blood-clotting mechanisms and blood pressure, decrease HDL (good), and increase LDL (bad) cholesterol levels and triglycerides, they can facilitate the development of insulin resistance and increase your risk of cardiovascular disease. These hormones and fatty acids are then released into the bloodstream and are directly transported to your liver, where they can interfere with insulin metabolism and create high insulin levels, poor blood sugar control, salt retention, high blood pressure, and inflammation.

Belly Fat and Diabetes/Insulin Resistance

Produced by the pancreas, insulin is a hormone that regulates blood sugar levels (glucose) and fat metabolism. Every time you eat, insulin is released to help your body use or store the glucose it gets from food. When men follow the typical American diet they eat highly processed foods that spike their blood sugars. These foods result in elevated levels of insulin that persist throughout the day, and their bodies begin to lose sensitivity to their own insulin. This causes insulin resistance—the first step toward type 2 diabetes. This type of diabetes is caused by poor nutrition and lack of exercise: As body fat levels increase, insulin sensitivity plummets.

Typical American Diet

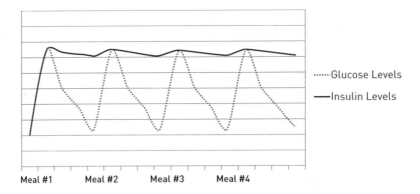

Glucose Levels
Insulin Levels

Meal #1   Meal #2   Meal #3   Meal #4

As insulin sensitivity drops, insulin secretion from your pancreas increases, triggering a multitude of changes, which include damage to the lining of your body's blood vessels (endothelial dysfunction). It also interferes with the enzymes that break down fats in your blood, and with your kidney's ability to get rid of sodium (causing high blood pressure). Insulin resistance is associated with chronically elevated levels of insulin and blood sugars (although blood sugars can be normal, especially early in the disease) and is present in most people with cardiovascular disease. High insulin levels also adversely affect your body fat percentage, aerobic capacity, muscle mass, strength, and immune function, all of which make it even more difficult to exercise. For all of these reasons, excess levels of insulin may be the single most important factor in accelerating the aging process.

Insulin not only promotes big bellies, but also prevents our fat cells from converting their stored fat into the free fatty acids that we can use for energy. Because we are unable to tap into this huge energy reservoir, we get tired and hungry between meals when our blood sugars are low, and we are subsequently driven to eat more sugar-rich foods to satisfy our energy needs. This promotes a vicious cycle of unstable blood sugars, elevated insulin levels, and uncontrolled eating, which persists and actually worsens over time. But when insulin levels are kept low you not only reduce your risk for both diabetes and heart disease, you are much less likely to convert calories into body fat. All insulin-related problems can be avoided by following my Life Plan Diet, which is specifically designed to keep blood sugars and insulin levels low.

Life Plan Diet

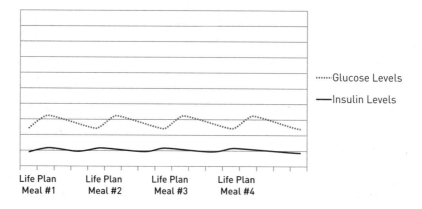

........Glucose Levels

——Insulin Levels

Life Plan Meal #1   Life Plan Meal #2   Life Plan Meal #3   Life Plan Meal #4

Another problem with living with elevated blood sugars is *glycation* (or glycosylation), the process in which glucose that's floating around in your bloodstream becomes attached to proteins and nucleic acids and produces new, very dangerous chemical structures. Ninety-nine percent of all cellular activities depend on the vast array of proteins in our bodies, and when sugars bind to them they become dysfunctional and create major problems. These glycated proteins are called *advanced glycation end-products* (AGEs), and they attack collagen, which is used to make ligaments, tendons, and other connective tissue important for muscle strength and growth, as well as nucleic acids, which are vital to the synthesis of new protein. Glycated proteins become very "sticky" and adhere to the inside walls of blood vessels, causing endothelial dysfunction, which leads to vascular dysfunction and arterial plaque. This then obstructs blood flow to the heart (leading to heart attacks), brain (causing strokes), and the hands, feet, eyes, muscles, and other vital organs. In extreme cases, a lack of blood flow to the extremities can necessitate amputation. Over time the function of all of our cells and arteries becomes seriously compromised, resulting in significant health consequences, including both mental and physical deterioration. Glycation is considered to be one of the most significant biological markers of aging. However, when glycation rates are controlled and kept low by the right nutrition, insulin levels are also kept low. Doctors can measure glycation by using a blood test called *hemoglobin A1c*. If you follow my specific nutritional recommendations in combination with my exercise program you can minimize glycation and add 10 to 15 years to your life. That is, 10 to 15 additional years of vitality, productivity, and great health—not 10 to 15 more years in a nursing home.

One of the major goals of this program is to enable you to increase your own production of the necessary male hormones, including human growth hormone (hGH). hGH is measured as IGF-1 (Insulin-like Growth Factor 1). As the name implies, Insulin-like Growth Factor 1 is structurally related to insulin. These two hormones share the same receptor sites on cells, creating a competition in which only one hormone will be predominantly effective. Because you need to optimize growth hormone levels to achieve great health and quality of life, my plan is designed to effectively manage your insulin, which will help you achieve healthy levels of growth hormone on your own. A nutrition program that focuses on keeping insulin levels as low as possible will enable you to increase your own natural production of IGF-1.

Controlling insulin levels is the primary objective of my nutrition plan, because it is the key to longevity and a disease-free life. This can best be achieved by eating small, frequent meals throughout the day and carefully limiting your carbohydrate choices to those with a low-glycemic index (mostly vegetables and nontropical fruits and only a few types of whole grains). It is also important to always eat a high-quality, low-fat source of protein with every carbohydrate.

A study in the *American Journal of Nutrition* compared diets with the same number of calories but different protein-to-carb ratios. The diet with a protein-to-carbohydrate ratio of 0.6 (similar to my Life Plan Diet) keeps insulin levels low and maintains a positive protein balance. The diets higher in carbohydrates and lower in protein, such as the American Heart Association Diet (with a protein-to-carbohydrate ratio of 0.25), tend to increase insulin secretion and produce a negative protein balance, allowing your body to begin breaking down your own muscle mass to provide energy for your body. That's why when you structure your nutrition program around keeping blood sugars and insulin levels in check and increasing protein you will get another big benefit—increased muscle size.

In just four to seven days of eating "clean" you will have your blood sugar and insulin levels in the ideal metabolic range, and by two weeks into the Life Plan Diet you will no longer be plagued by feelings of fatigue, hunger, deprivation, and cravings. You'll experience a marked improvement in your mental focus, exercise endurance, strength, and leanness. When your body fat disappears and your muscle mass increases, your insulin resistance will also diminish, taking a huge burden off your pancreas so that it can now secrete less insulin throughout the day. What's more, the greater your insulin sensitivity, the more effective you become at removing sugar from your blood and tapping into your fat stores for your energy needs, leading to even more belly fat loss. *It's physiologically impossible for you to burn your body fat for energy when your insulin levels are high.* You'll also reduce your desire for consuming extra calories, because your body can now tap into stored body fat more efficiently. You literally become a fat-burning machine!

Belly Fat and Inflammation

Inflammation is the body's way of initiating healing. It is a complex biological response of vascular tissues to harmful stimulants or irritants. The classic signs of inflammation are pain, redness, and swelling, which occur as a protective attempt to remove injurious stimuli from the organ they are attacking. For example, when you have an allergic reaction, the vascular tissues in your eyes and nose may swell up, causing pain (headache) and redness in the eyes. However, when you remove the offending allergen, the inflammation ceases.

Inflammation that is unregulated can result in excessive internal activity and tissue destruction, which can lead to a host of diseases. This type of chronic inflammation can occur only internally, and you may never realize that it is taking place. That's why chronic inflammation is often referred to as "silent inflammation." This insidious form of inflammation is thought to be at the root of all of the age-related diseases, and is caused by prolonged levels of elevated insulin, which you now know occur with carrying around excess fat. The men whom I see in my practice who have elevated inflammatory markers all have big bellies, and as I said earlier, their belly fat itself is causing this continuing inflammation.

The good news is that the fix is relatively easy. By reducing belly fat through diet you will reduce insulin resistance and thereby inflammation. Then you will be able to dramatically slow the aging process and prevent or reverse serious disease. The best way to decrease the production of insulin is by following a noninflammatory, low-glycemic diet that controls insulin production, like the one in this book, which is rich in lean proteins, omega-3 fatty acids, antioxidants, and minerals. These include colorful vegetables, brown rice, yams, and sprouted grain breads.

Belly Fat and Heart Disease

When we compare the types of body fat on men to women, men have close to twice the amount of belly fat. It's been hypothesized that this difference in the location of body fat is the primary reason that heart disease is more prevalent—and more deadly—in men than in women. If your waistline is greater than 35 inches measured just above your belly button, you're at a higher risk for developing two or more risk factors for heart disease. These include glucose intolerance (elevated levels of blood sugar), insulin resistance, dyslipidemia (abnormal cholesterol—low HDL and high LDL—and high triglycerides), hypertension, and inflammation. The reason that I'm so committed to treating men before they develop any of these risk factors is that the number-one symptom of heart disease is sudden death.

Inflammation is intrinsically connected to all phases of cardiovascular disease. One serious outcome of inflammation is atherosclerosis (plaque buildup), which occurs when artery walls thicken as a result of the accumulation of fatty materials such as cholesterol and triglycerides. Atherosclerosis is a chronic response that involves an increase in inflammatory white blood cells, which is promoted by an increase of LDL or "bad" cholesterol and a decrease of HDL or "good" cholesterol. Atherosclerosis can begin in childhood as a result of damage to the endothelium (the thin lining of the arteries). Most heart attacks and strokes occur when a blood clot forms in inflamed plaque, cutting off the blood supply to the affected heart or brain tissue. The fatter you are in and around your waist, the more likely this is to happen, because of the chronic inflammation you are producing in your blood vessels.

Take my experience as an example. When I was 60 I learned that I had advanced, chronic heart disease involving my coronary arteries, which began back in my 20s. According to my cardiologist, what saved me from an early death was my wife, Annie, motivating me to enter the Body-*for*-LIFE contest, along with the healthy aging program I have been following ever since: a combination of low-glycemic, low-fat nutrition; supplements; a vital exercise regimen; and correcting my hormone deficiencies. This combination helped me get rid of my gut so that I was able to decrease inflammation and stabilize my heart disease. I've learned over the past 16 years that everything I put in my mouth can either heal me or kill me. Knowing this has totally changed my attitude about food and drink. Now it's much easier for me to make the right choices so that I don't continue to form plaque and promote silent inflammation that could lead to a heart attack or stroke. If I had known the importance of making good, healthy food choices when I was in my 40s, I would have been able to totally prevent my coronary artery disease. The program that I'm outlining in this book will guide you along the path of healthy eating that I wish I had known about and started decades ago. You'll have the knowledge I was missing, and you will avoid ending up among the 70 percent of men who die of heart disease prematurely simply because they have made bad lifestyle choices. Heart disease may still take me out of this world, but I definitely know that if it does, I have delayed it by many years as a result of all the healthy things I promote in my books and on my website.

Belly Fat and Metabolic Syndrome

Metabolic syndrome occurs when your excess weight affects all of the above-mentioned conditions. It is a cluster of abnormalities that include high blood pressure, increased blood sugar, excess belly fat, and abnormal cholesterol levels. These conditions occur simultaneously, increasing your risk for diabetes, heart disease, stroke, cancer, and Alzheimer's disease (all of the age-related diseases). Metabolic syndrome is also linked to sexual dysfunction.

However, metabolic syndrome is completely and totally preventable and reversible. Weight loss, exercise, and correcting hormone deficiencies are the keys to preventing this disease as well as losing body fat—especially belly fat.

Belly Fat and Asthma, Snoring, and Sleep Apnea

A recent Mayo Clinic study has linked sleep deprivation to obesity. The study found that people who achieved fewer than five hours of sleep a night consumed 549 additional calories during the day. In another 2012 study published in the *Journal of Clinical Endocrinology & Metabolism*, it was shown that a poor night's sleep can activate the appetite-controlling part of the brain, increasing levels of hunger throughout the day. We also know that being overweight is one of the causes of sleep apnea, which can disturb sleep patterns all night long.

Men who have large bellies have trouble breathing day and night. This is because they have difficulty moving their diaphragm, a sheet of internal skeletal muscle that extends across the bottom of the rib cage and separates the thoracic cavity (which contains the heart, lungs, and ribs) from the abdominal cavity. The diaphragm is where respiration occurs: As the diaphragm contracts, the volume of the thoracic cavity increases and air is drawn into the lungs. But when your belly is full of fat, your diaphragm cannot move down to expand your lungs, and this obviously interferes with your ability to breathe. You end up taking shorter, shallower breaths, which inhibit your ability to fully oxygenate your blood and send oxygen to all your vital organs. The buildup of belly fat is a very slow process, so men don't realize their ability to take air into their lungs is impaired. Most will attribute their shortness of breath to aging, or being "out of shape," but not to their belly fat. I should also point out that it really doesn't take much belly fat (5 to 10 pounds) to profoundly affect your ability to breathe. Just carrying an extra five pounds will cause me to feel short of breath, and I'm in excellent athletic shape.

This whole disturbance is analogous to women during pregnancy, who have trouble taking in enough air. But pregnancy is a temporary condition that ends as soon as the baby is delivered. Pregnant women know why they are short of breath; most men with belly fat don't. Men who carry around belly fat can't resolve poor breathing habits, and in fact, their breathing gets worse as they gain more weight. These are the folks who are likely to be hospitalized for asthma and other respiratory problems. A 2003 study in the journal *Chest* reported that 75 percent of patients treated for asthma at the emergency room were overweight or obese. What's more, abdominal obesity affecting pulmonary function occurs more often in men than in women.

The same problem occurs at night, with potentially more devastating results. Obstructive Sleep Apnea Syndrome (OSAS) is another breathing problem that affects overweight men. If you have been told that you snore loudly, wake up in the middle of the night gasping for air, or feel constantly fatigued in the morning, you may have OSAS. Sleep apnea refers to the phenomenon of sudden breathing interruptions during sleep. It disrupts the stage of sleep in which you experience rapid eye movement (REM) and prevents you from attaining a good night's rest. In the worst case, it can kill you, because you are depriving your brain of the proper levels of oxygen. During sleep, when oxygen levels naturally start to decline, people with sleep apnea lose the automatic stimulus to keep breathing. When this happens, oxygen levels drop and carbon dioxide levels increase, which forces breathing in short bursts that can be violent enough to wake you up.

Sleep apnea occurs when two different issues converge: poor sleep position and excess body fat. Together these cause airway blockage in both the chest and the neck, resulting in both snoring and sleep apnea. The greater the blockages, the louder men snore, and at the same time, the blockages lower the air volume as well as overall oxygen levels in the blood.

Many overweight men are most comfortable sleeping on their back, causing additional pressure on the diaphragm, which interferes with their breathing. Sleep apnea can be resolved by using an external CPAP machine, which forces air and oxygen into the lungs all night long. If you already use a CPAP, continue to use it while you lose your belly fat. Once you've lost the weight, get another sleep study and you may be pleasantly surprised that you don't need it anymore.

Belly Fat and Sexual Dysfunction

The absolute most important component in my mind to sexual dysfunction is belly fat. When men successfully lose belly fat their self-image improves, and their performance improves. However, there are also some physiological reasons why men have problems with their sexual function. Although the public is vastly more educated about erectile dysfunction, or ED, thanks to those ubiquitous ads, many men are still embarrassed by their lack of performance and hesitant to talk to their doctors. Yet it's critical that you do address the issue head-on, because, aside from living with a disappointing sex life, your sexual function is actually a window into your total health. Your ability to maintain an erection and achieve orgasm on an average of three times a week is a key benchmark that you're healthy and physically fit.

Erectile dysfunction, which is defined as the persistent inability to attain or maintain an erection, affects over 30 million American men, an estimated 34 percent of men age 40 to 70. It is directly associated with cardiovascular disease, hypertension, diabetes, and metabolic syndrome. In fact, one of the first signs of heart disease is a reduction in penile hardness. An August 2010 study in the *Journal of Sexual Medicine* showed that typically men begin having ED issues four to five years before their first heart attack.

Erectile dysfunction is directly connected to another type of "ED," this time concerning the endothelium, the lining of your blood vessels, which is associated with circulation. Endothelial dysfunction can be the first rung of the atherosclerosis ladder, leading to heart disease and stroke. The penis is actually composed of an extensive endothelial surface interlaced with smooth muscle. Atherosclerosis (plaque buildup in your arteries) can occur throughout the body. So if the arteries supplying your heart with blood have atherosclerosis—or heart disease—it's not surprising that the smaller arteries of your penis are affected. For that matter, because of their size, the arteries of the penis narrow sooner than the arteries to your heart. This is exactly why ED is an early warning sign for heart disease and may be a predictive sign of stroke later in life.

But before you start popping those little blue pills, take off a few pounds. Close to 80 percent of men with moderate to severe erection problems are overweight or obese, which leads to the silent inflammation we discussed earlier. Although this time it's not so silent, because when the penile arteries are inflamed, they interfere with the blood supply to the penis, and that's something to shout about, although most guys, unfortunately, keep quiet about it.

A second concern is the basic mechanics of sex. A man's big, pregnantlike belly can make sexual intercourse much more challenging and less enjoyable for both you and your partner. As you slim down, you'll also feel more limber and flexible. And as my Pilates instructor still likes to say, "A flexible man is a sexual man."

Abdominal obesity is also correlated with low testosterone levels, which adds to any man's sexual function issues. Testosterone is the male sex hormone responsible for your favorite pastime, and I'm not referring to baseball or fishing. You simply can't have sex without testosterone. But you might not know that it is also very necessary for maintaining high energy levels and vitality, increasing your muscle mass and overall strength (men simply can't build muscle without it), enhancing your ability to burn body fat (especially around and inside the waist), improving your mood and emotional well-being, preventing bone loss, keeping your mind sharp, and protecting your heart. Without testosterone you cannot lose weight. And when you are overly fat your ability to make your own testosterone becomes impaired. In fact, belly fat tissue produces estrogen, which competes with and inhibits testosterone production and causes the dreaded "man boobs."

An important and often overlooked cause of decreased testosterone levels is chronic emotional stress. The continued release of stress hormones such as cortisol severely inhibits testosterone production. For all men age 30 and older, testosterone begins to drop 1 to 3 percent annually. Because the drop is slow and steady, symptoms of low testosterone are sometimes imperceptible until bigger health problems emerge. Around age 40, the drop increases, and you will begin to notice. By your mid-40s, you start complaining about "feeling older." As a result, your work productivity declines, and you worry about the competition from the younger guys in the office. And as I experienced, your once-effective workout won't deliver the same results.

One of the telltale indicators of low-T is a lack in frequency of early morning erections and spontaneous erections. With lowered testosterone, not only do early morning erections disappear, but erectile performance, libido, and sexual thoughts throughout the day also take a hit. Here are some other signs that your levels are falling, and as you'll see, they are very similar to the list of symptoms related to being overly fat. This is one of the reasons why low-T and weight gain are interrelated:

- Declining sexual and physical energy
- Disturbed sleep
- Emotional swings, irritability, anxiety, depression
- Foggy thinking, memory lapses
- Increased cardiovascular issues
- Loss of strength
- Poor skin tone and saggy, wrinkled skin
- Reduced lean muscle, higher body fat
- Weak bones, osteopenia, osteoporosis

However, the right fat-loss plan can address your symptoms. Penile hardness tests have shown that men having the best sexual performance:

- Are in excellent health
- Don't smoke or drink

- Eat clean

- Get plenty of rest

- Exercise frequently

- Maintain optimal hormone levels

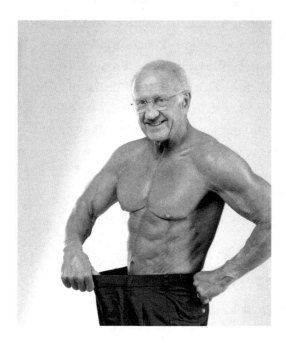

What's Your Current Health Status?

The first step to any program is to create a baseline in order to chart your improvement. Answer the following questions. If you answer "yes" to any of them you know that your waistline is negatively affecting your overall health. Then, see a doctor before starting the Life Plan Diet so that you can work together and chart a course of action. Once a month, return to this questionnaire and see how your health has improved as you begin to lose not only pounds, but inches.

1. Is your pants size larger than when you graduated from high school?

2. Do you have difficulty tying your shoes?

3. Can you buy a suit "off the rack" without having the waistline taken in? (Off-the-rack suits are tailored for "the average guy," and we know that average guys in this country are overweight or just too fat and die of heart disease.)

4. When you stand naked with your back, shoulders, and butt placed firmly against a wall and look down, is your penis blocked from your view?

5. Are you short of breath after climbing one flight of stairs?

6. Does your belly interfere with sexual intercourse?

7. From a standing position and with your knees locked, can you touch your toes?

8. Do you use most of the seat belt or require an extender when flying?

9. Do you frequently get cravings for high-sugar or high-fat food?

10. Do you wake up tired and dread getting out of bed to start your day?

11. Do you have problems walking in airports faster than other people?

12. Do you feel old?

13. Does your profile photo resemble that of a woman in the final term of pregnancy?

14. Have you been told that you would make an excellent Santa Claus by friends or relatives?

15. Do you avoid being seen in a bathing suit without a shirt?

The good news is that even a small weight loss (between 5 and 10 percent of your current weight) will help lower your risk of developing all of these health issues. With proper nutrition, the right kind of exercise, and healthy hormone levels, you'll be able not only to reverse disease but improve your quality of life now and going forward. You can plan for a future of good health, but you have to start the hard work right now. Now let's see how your weight is affecting your thinking, your mood, and the way you're dealing with others.

CHAPTER 2

Slim Down to Stay Smart and Calm

New scientific breakthroughs regarding brain health have been extensively reported in the news recently, and for good reason. Every day, researchers are uncovering more information about how the brain works and what the best courses of action should be in order to keep your mind functioning optimally for as long as possible. That's a particularly important goal: Alzheimer's disease and dementia are among the biggest fears people have when it comes to their health. In fact, the majority of men are more afraid of losing their minds than they are of developing cancer.

The brain is considered to be the final frontier of modern medicine. Diagnostic imaging allows researchers previously unheard-of access to the living brain in order to have a better understanding of how it functions in real time. New discoveries provide insight into how we create and store memories; how mood affects learning; and how the brain controls not only what we think about but how we feel, as well as our physical health. Perhaps the most significant finding is that if the brain is properly nourished it can continue to grow new brain cells even as we age. This concept is called *neurogenesis*, and it means that we are not destined to a life of forgetfulness as we get older. In fact, each new brain cell guarantees that we can continue to learn new skills and keep the ones we have well into the future.

At this point you might be thinking that I've lost my mind and wandered off onto some weird tangent that has nothing to do with diet. But the truth is that your weight and your overall health directly affect brain function, and vice versa. When you are in good physical health, your cognition—the speed at which you think and pay attention and your ability to remember—can remain at peak levels even as you age. This idea has been around for some time, but many discarded it as the wishful thinking of preventive medicine specialists like me. Now, however, science is on our side. Two groundbreaking studies released in 2013 confirm what I have been preaching: that proactively ensuring optimal health through lifestyle modification can lead to a decreased risk of dementia, not only now, but as you age. The studies showed that the incidence of dementia is lower among those who control their blood pressure and cholesterol, possibly because some dementia is caused by mini strokes and other vascular damage. The populations that were able to control cardiovascular risk factors better through diet and exercise were the least likely to succumb.

This brand-new research points to the fact that you are in charge of your future. If you believe that you're not thinking as clearly as you used to, it's not simply a sign of normal aging that you have to live with. Instead, it's a wakeup call for you to take a good look at how your health is affecting your thinking. Your expanding waistline is not only making your body sick and old, it is limiting your ability to grow new brain cells and negatively affecting your vascular network, both of which are increasing your chances of developing dementia.

Again, this isn't a best-guess analysis: It's real science. A study in the March 2009 issue of *Archives of Neurology* investigated whether total and/or regional body fat levels influence cognitive decline. Researchers found that in men, worsening cognitive function correlated with the highest levels of all adiposity measures: The fatter you are, the more likely you will experience cognitive decline later in life. In one study it was found that obesity was associated with an almost tenfold increased risk of ending up with Alzheimer's disease.

Once you add in factors like metabolic syndrome, the risk of developing dementia and Alzheimer's disease is even higher. People with diabetes are at least twice as likely to get Alzheimer's, and while diabetes doesn't "cause" Alzheimer's, these two diseases may have the same root: an overconsumption of foods that mess with insulin and blood sugar control. In other words, when you have abdominal obesity and other metabolic issues going on, such as insulin resistance and elevated cholesterol levels, your risk of developing Alzheimer's is even greater.

And just as I mentioned in the last chapter, where you carry your extra weight matters. Another study reported in 2010 in the *Annals of Neurology*, examining more than

700 adults, found evidence to suggest that higher volumes of belly fat, regardless of overall weight, were associated with smaller brain volumes and increased risk of dementia. Hmmm, the bigger your belly the smaller your brain. Maybe my brain has gotten bigger since my "before" picture at age 57!

Symptoms of a Failing Brain

You know when you're sharp as a tack, ready to take on the world, and when you are not. Many experts refer to less effective thinking as *brain fog*. This can include feeling spaced out, forgetful, confused, lost, and tired and having difficulty with concentration. If you're not keeping up in the office or you're slow to remember where you're supposed to be, you may be experiencing brain fog, which is considered to be among the first signs of mild cognitive impairment, or worse: the initial stages of early-onset Alzheimer's disease.

However, it's important to distinguish between normal memory lapses and significant memory problems such as Alzheimer's disease, which typically affect multiple aspects of daily life. As the Alzheimer's Association points out, if you forget where you put your keys, that's a problem with memory that can be related to stress or anxiety. If you forget what keys are for, that's a sign that you are heading toward dementia and Alzheimer's disease.

Luckily, just as you can proactively take care of your body, you can also provide the optimal nourishment for your brain so that you can prevent, and even reverse, poor brain health. Best of all, taking care of your brain does not require much more effort than taking care of your body. The same methods you'll use to slim down, including choosing the right foods, engaging in exercise, and correcting hormone deficiencies, can help you avoid brain fog so that you can think clearly for the rest of your life.

Taking a Load Off Your Brain

Even the best diet and exercise regimen on the planet wouldn't be enough to keep your brain and body healthy if you don't manage stress levels first. Stress can actually reshape the brain. While the right amount of stress is beneficial and necessary for neuronal growth, severe or chronic stress can be harmful and cause long-lasting damage, affecting behavior, learning, and memory. In this way the health of your brain directly affects the health of your body.

For many men, stress leads directly to weight gain. There are a handful of reasons why this occurs: First, when we're stressed, our attention and ability to make good decisions diminish, and we are prone to make bad food choices. We look for foods that are expedient and available rather than what will be good for our bodies in the long run. These bad choices are typically simple carbohydrates that actually do make you feel better, yet when combined with excess cortisol, can also make you retain fluid and feel bloated.

The go-to choice for "self-medicating" stress tends to be carbohydrate binges: comfort foods and alcohol. A British study found that men with job stress were nearly twice as likely to develop metabolic syndrome as their unstressed peers. While you may feel calmer in the short run after a couple of drinks or a plate of lasagna, you are also causing insulin resistance and weight gain with these poor choices. Your body just can't handle the crap that you are eating.

When I was younger and had had a really rough day at work, I'd come home and try to relax with a drink or two or three. I didn't know that I was making that specific choice because my attention to my own health was diminished: I simply couldn't concentrate on making a good choice because I just wanted to relax. But today, when I have the same bad day, I make a better choice and go straight to my exercise bike to relieve the stress. By the time I get off, I feel great: reenergized and relaxed. What I've been able to do is readdress my attention toward something that is ultimately positive for my health (exercise) rather than something negative (alcohol) in order to lighten my stress levels. Instead of stuffing yourself with beer, vodka, chips, or doughnuts, the Life Plan Diet will help you kick those habits and empower you to choose foods that will calm the brain as well as satisfy your stomach.

A second factor is the body's response to stress. As we learned in Chapter 1, if your mental state is overwhelmed by stress—from work, your home life, your health, or other past traumas—both your body and your brain react by reducing the effectiveness of all the less-than-vital systems, including digestion and attention. Traffic, a hard workday, or living with chronic pain can instigate a stress response that can impair your body's ability to move on to normal functions in both the short and long term, also leading to weight gain.

Diet and Exercise Reduce Stress and Improve Brain Health

Most American men participate in this stress loop every single day of their lives. Eating or drinking your way out of stress with comfort foods and alcohol will only spike your blood sugar and insulin levels and cause inflammation to skyrocket, which just adds more stress to what your body is already experiencing. This cycle has got to be stopped, because it will accelerate you down the path to all the diseases mentioned in Chapter 1 as well as Alzheimer's. In other words, it puts you on course to getting old very fast.

The best foods to choose when you are stressed are not high-glycemic carbs, but rather protein and low-glycemic carbohydrates such as brown rice or yams. The right proteins keep you feeling full so that hunger doesn't add to your stress level. Low-glycemic carbs provide you with a slow, steady state of sugar released into your bloodstream, which is your brain's main source of energy. This helps you think more clearly and make better decisions about how you'll deal with your stress.

Making sure that you have enough calories during the day is another way to lower stress. When the brain starts to feel that it is getting low on fuel it drives you to find a quick source, usually in the form of high-glycemic carbohydrates, which we experience as food cravings. At the same time the brain forces what we call a *starvation response*, which causes the immediate storage of food as body fat so that it will be available to the brain at another time. This strategy works for the brain, but not for the belly. However, once you start feeding your brain regularly with good food choices, you will start dropping pounds of belly fat.

There are even better ways to reduce stress without resorting to food and drink. Aerobic exercise, which burns up cortisol and releases endorphins, delivers almost instantaneous stress relief and is a great coping strategy to help you cut loose from everyday pressures. Endorphins are brain chemicals that are similar to the prescription drug morphine. When they are released they can help relieve pain and make us feel good. They provide us with a positive outlook on life without leading to addiction or chemical dependence.

I also find that stretching helps relieve the tension that builds in my body throughout the day. Exercise can promote an overall pattern of calmness in certain parts of the brain, reducing anxiety. This is accomplished through the release of GABA, a brain chemical that promotes a relaxation response.

We also know that exercise promotes neurogenesis. One 2010 study from the Salk

Institute connects exercise to enhancing stem cell production in the brain, which is how new neurons are created. In animal studies, mice and rats that run for a few weeks generally show twice as many new neurons in their hippocampi as sedentary animals. Exercise also seems to make these new neurons nimble so that they can more easily connect into the neural network.

According to *Canyon Ranch 30 Days to a Better Brain*, exercise may be one of the best things you can do for your brain, because it has been directly correlated with protecting and improving brain health, as well as enhancing cognitive performance. Beginning in our late 20s, most of us will annually lose about 1 percent of the volume of the hippocampus, a key portion of the brain related to memory and learning. Exercise seems to slow or reverse the brain's decay, much as it does with muscles. In a 2011 study released from the University of Arizona, researchers found that physically fit older men and women show fewer age-related changes in their brains. The study showed that regular exercise was crucial in preserving key parts of the brain involved in attention and memory. The more physically fit individuals were, the fewer age-related brain changes the researchers could find. And for people who have already experienced losses in cognitive function, exercise has also been a key feature in reversing poor brain health. A 2010 study from the University of Washington School of Medicine documented that in as little as six months exercise improves cognitive performance in older adults with mild cognitive impairment.

One of the most effective techniques to reduce and manage chronic stress is cognitive-behavioral therapy. This includes identifying the sources of stress in your life, restructuring your priorities, changing your response to stress, and finally, finding methods to manage and reduce or totally eliminate the stress. You may need to work with a psychologist who is well trained in cognitive-behavioral therapy to develop the skills you need to manage your stress. This will not only improve your life but will help you gain control over your eating.

Eliminate Emotional Eating

The real secret to losing weight, and keeping it off forever, is to recognize when you are eating because you are hungry, and when you are eating as a way to fill a void. This type of eating is called *emotional eating*. Most men disregard emotional eating as a women's issue, but I find that men are just as likely to do this, because they have a harder time dealing with their emotions over the course of the day than women do. They subsequently deal with their issues with food and, more often than not, alcohol.

Emotional eating can occur at any time—during meals, at the end of meals, between meals, at social occasions, and late at night. One of the biggest battles that I have had to deal with over the past 16 years is cravings that begin after I've eaten the last meal of the day. My days at work are particularly stressful, and there have been many nights when I couldn't fall asleep until I ate something that would raise my blood sugars to unacceptably high levels. This is definitely not the way to get rid of belly fat, and I'm sure it increased my risk for advancing coronary artery disease. The way I finally broke this habit was to make my final meal of the day one cup of frozen black seedless grapes. For me, this does the trick, because I end the day with something that satisfies my sweet tooth yet has only 60 calories and is still considered to be low-glycemic. The key for me is to make sure that I don't eat too many, and these grapes have to be frozen, because when they are, I can't eat them very fast or have very many.

For me, the secret was to meet my needs with a healthy alternative. You will have to figure out your own strategy to handle your particular cravings. But the key to curing yourself of all bad habits is to not give in to them. Don't have unhealthy foods in the house and you won't think about them nearly as often. The longer you can stay away from your particular demon foods, the less you will think about them and want them.

The most common reasons for emotional eating are typically negative experiences, which can include:

- Anger
- Anxiety
- Boredom
- Fear
- Depression
- Hurt feelings
- Loneliness
- Stress
- Turmoil arising from childhood trauma

Positive emotions can be emotional-eating triggers as well. When you step out for a celebratory lunch with your office staff, or take your wife or partner out for an anniversary dinner, you are creating new triggers for food built around happy occasions. The trick to breaking this cycle is to think of other ways to reward yourself that don't involve food.

The first step toward eliminating emotional eating is to make eating a more conscious activity. Eating must always be organized and well planned. I don't recommend eating at your desk, in your car as you're rushing from one activity to another, or while you watch TV. This kind of eating is mindless. You can't enjoy the food you are eating and send satiety signals to your brain if you are doing two things at once, so you just continue to feel hungry and anxious even as you are eating.

Instead, take the time to sit down at a table and really enjoy your food, even if you are by yourself. The meals on the Life Plan Diet won't take long to prepare, and they certainly won't take a long time to eat. Make sure you eat slowly, chew your food thoroughly, and savor every bite. By setting aside this time and focusing on your food, you are adding appreciation to your meal and the whole process of eating. This helps me reduce the anxiety that I have created over the years surrounding my relationship with food, because in the moment I'm able to take the pressure off of myself and simply focus on enjoying the meal.

Next, let's work on distinguishing the point where physical hunger ends and emotional eating begins. Most of us in America rarely experience real physical hunger, because food is so plentiful and available. We operate almost exclusively off of emotional hunger, or we eat by the clock. I have learned that when I'm really hungry I feel it throughout my body. My energy levels decline, I get a feeling of massive fatigue, and my muscles begin to ache. I feel the urgent need to eat a healthy, balanced meal, which corrects all of this within a few minutes.

Some men tell me that they get a headache when they are hungry. Others confuse hunger with thirst. Whatever your reaction, once you've identified it, you can begin the hard work of taking a clear and objective look and start making the changes needed for permanently eliminating emotional eating so that you eat only when you are really hungry. And don't forget, real hunger is a great sign that you are in a caloric deficit and burning body fat. Even when you follow this diet and you are eating every two to three hours, try to wait until you begin to feel hungry before you start your next meal.

Track your hunger by keeping a food journal, like the one I provide in Appendix A. By writing down how you feel after every meal, as well as exactly what you ate, you'll learn to distinguish between eating emotionally and eating because you are really hungry.

The successful elimination of this destructive behavior might require making significant changes in your life. These changes can be as simple as developing creative ways to handle stress, or as involved as entering a psychological counseling program. Whatever they are, you'll find that you are going to be much more successful following this diet once you take control of how and when you eat.

Food Addiction Starts in the Brain

Just as people with food allergies know that they can't eat certain foods or they will have a reaction, you may have the same relationship with certain foods, only the reaction is that they cause you to eat more. We all have our own "trigger foods" that cause us to binge beyond our hunger. These cravings are the first and most important sign that you may have a food addiction.

It's quite rare for Brussels sprouts, chicken, broccoli, and asparagus to fall into the trigger food category. Instead, chronic exposure to foods high in combinations of sugar, fat, and salt can rewire the brain to promote and amplify this craving mechanism. Dr. Ann Kelly from the University of Wisconsin authored a study showing that fat is highly addictive, especially when you add sugar or salt to it, making your favorite potato chips or French fries the "perfect storm" of food addiction. These foods are thought to stimulate the same circuits in the brain that are activated by pleasure-producing, mind-altering drugs or other addictive behavior, such as sex. In fact, many researchers believe trigger foods invoke a loss of control that duplicates the behavioral consequences of addiction.

The desire for a particular food, or what we refer to as cravings, signals the release of the brain chemical dopamine. A 2005 landmark study by Drs. Nora Volkow and Roy Wise determined that the brain responds to food in the same way it responds to heavily addictive drugs such as cocaine. If you experience food cravings and find that you need more of a particular food each time you eat it in order to feel satisfied, you may be addicted to food.

A true food addiction doesn't mean you need two cookies at the end of a meal to feel satisfied: That's a learned behavioral response, or a habit. Instead, an addiction occurs when you think you are going to eat two cookies, but in five minutes you've wolfed down the whole package. An alcohol addiction isn't the ritual of having one martini when you get home from work, but having three or four with dinner. However, you will need to break both addictions and bad eating habits, because even two cookies a day, or that one perfect martini, signals some form of self-medicating with food that will ultimately sabotage your efforts to get rid of your belly.

The only way to maintain control over trigger foods and food addictions is by totally avoiding them. Don't deceive yourself: You will never be able to control a trigger food. The idea that you can have just "a little" never works! This is why 95 percent of dieters who are able to lose fat gain it all back in 12 to 18 months. When people reach their goal weight most of them think they have gained control over their trigger foods. But trigger foods always win. You can never control them.

Some of us may be genetically predisposed to reduced dopamine levels, making us even more susceptible to overconsumption/addictive behavior. But there's hope. You can rewire your circuitry and reboot your brain as I did to beat addiction and feel better than ever. If avoidance isn't enough to quash your cravings and you find yourself yearning for your favorite trigger foods, you may need to seek professional help. Don't despair: With the proper care, which may include medication and counseling, most men can beat food addictions, just as I did.

The first step in successfully dealing with addictive behavior is to recognize that you have it. Review these signs and symptoms to determine if you may have a food addiction. If you answer "true" to more than four of these statements, discuss the outcome with your doctor, as well as the specific issues that triggered your positive response.

SIGNS OF A FOOD ADDICTION

1. When food, eating, or my weight becomes the topics of discussion, I withdraw or attempt to change the subject. T/F

2. There is at least one type of food I must eat every day. T/F

3. I use food as a way to deal with my emotions. T/F

4. I often eat in front of the TV, or graze mindlessly throughout the day. T/F

5. I spend time every day buying food for myself or my family. T/F

6. I know I eat far more than I need of certain foods, but it makes me feel better to eat it, even when I'm not hungry. T/F

7. I feel powerless when I have a craving. T/F

8. I often feel sluggish after I eat. T/F

9. I can't go to bed without having a late-night sweet snack. T/F

10. My favorite foods include doughnuts, ice cream, French fries, cookies, breakfast cereals, or chips. T/F

Once you determine which foods are addictive for you, treat them like heroin—something that you know is especially dangerous—and completely avoid them. This means never tempt or convince yourself that you can try to go back and eat or drink in a controlled way. There is no such thing as a "free day" when it comes to avoiding these foods. It takes about a week of strict avoidance before cravings go away, and it may feel like the longest week of your life. But once the cravings are gone you will never have to worry about them again—unless you go back. If you do, you'll find that it can take days, and even weeks, to get yourself back on track.

Overcoming addictions is hard work. I know that it takes time, persistence, and a single-minded approach. Over the past 16 years I have had great success in controlling my own destructive addictions—food and alcohol. My secret has been to replace them with what I consider to be healthy addictions (exercise, especially cardio, clean eating, music, massage, stress-reducing strategies, etc.). Not every day has been perfect, and the journey has not always been easy. However, I'm much better off today than I was for the majority of my life, and I know that if I can master my addictions, so can you.

Now it's time to start your journey. In the next chapter, you'll learn how to determine how much fat you have to lose and how to track your success.

CHAPTER 3

Setting Goals and Changing Perceptions

The hallmark of a man who's in control of his body and his health is a strong, lean, ripped abdomen: That's the ultimate goal of this book. If you've talked to your doctor, he or she may have a specific weight-loss goal in mind. You might have a photo of when you were looking your best, from a wedding or family affair. Or, you might just remember how you used to feel and want to recapture that state of health.

My challenge to you is the same one I give all of my patients, including those who are already obese and affected by disease. I would like you to stay on this program forever, of course, but your primary objective is to get your waistline measurement down to 34 inches or less. Remember that belly fat is the first place you gain . . . and the last place you drop the weight. But don't get discouraged, because you can get rid of this stubborn belly fat, just as I have.

I'd also like to see you attain a percent body fat of 15 percent of your total weight or less. Body fat of more than 20 percent puts men in the over-fat, high-health-risk category. As a general rule, I believe no man at any age should have greater than 15 percent body fat if he wants to remain optimally fit and healthy. If it's a six-pack or a washboard stomach that you're after, you're going to have to lower your percent body fat down to less than 10 percent.

In the following table, I have listed the percentages of body fat for men according to their age that correlate with excellent to poor health/fitness ratings. You'll see that I've set the bar high for you: I'm not looking for "average" results. Average men die of heart disease. If you want to be able to live like a younger man, you have to work at keeping yourself slim. However, I can tell you firsthand that it's definitely worth the effort. At age 75, I work very hard at keeping my body fat below 10 percent, and at this percentage, I feel the best, have far greater energy, move better, think better, look my best, and have the lowest risk for disease and greater sexual function.

PERCENTAGE OF BODY FAT FOR MEN

Health/Fitness Rating	Age in years 20–29	Age in years 30–39	Age in years 40–49	Age in years 50–59	Age in years 60+
Excellent	<11	<12	<14	<15	<16
Good	11–13	12–14	14–16	15–17	16–18
Average	14–20	15–21	17–23	18–24	19–25
Fair	21–23	22–24	24–26	25–27	26–28
Poor	>23	>24	>26	>27	>28

Old Muscles Weigh Less, Not More

The typical middle-aged male—we're talking 50 on up—loses muscle mass (sarcopenia) and some bone mass (osteoporosis), which means that the weight of his muscles declines. This would lead you to think that men should lose weight as they age, but your own belly tells a different story. In fact, the average man's overall weight tends to go up as he ages, because he's adding more body fat on a less stable frame. This combination means that not only are men typically heavier as they age, they also become more flabby and frail. For some men, this decline can start as early as age 30. That's why you can't wait until you've fallen and broken a rib or an arm to start regaining muscle mass: If you're not building muscle mass, you're losing it.

Muscle is also the generator for your metabolism. As you lose muscle mass you're doing your own metabolism a disservice because you're decreasing its capacity. This is just another reason why you might weigh more than you did 10 years ago, even if you've been eating the same types of food. Declining hormone levels also contribute to decreasing metabolism.

If you've bought into the notion that as you age your whole body is going to slow down and you need to start taking it easy, you're setting yourself up for a situation where your own retirement is what's going to kill you. As soon as you stop moving you begin to gain body fat, even though you probably attribute your weight gain to the fact that you're getting older. The fact is that it's really not any harder for me to maintain or drop body fat at age 75 than it was at age 50 or 45, as long as I stay active. So stop making excuses: Men, you need to get it out of your head that getting fatter is part of the aging process, and that it's okay. It's not okay, unless you think getting age-related disease is okay.

Measure Your Gut

First, you need to know your baseline weight. Simple enough: Step on a scale without any clothes, first thing in the morning right after you get out of bed and go to the bathroom. This is because you weigh less in the morning, and when you weigh yourself the same way every time, you can develop a consistent and accurate reading of your weight.

While chronicling the pounds you shed is important, we're really more interested in measuring how much body fat you are losing. This story is told by the number of inches you can slice off your waist, as well as the ratio between your waist and the rest of you.

There are lots of fancy ways to assess your weight-loss goals, but the absolute best way is to simply take a couple of pictures of yourself. You need to strip down to a pair of shorts and have someone take two photographs of you without sucking in your gut. You'll need a shot of your front, and a second one that's a side view. Then, print out a couple of copies of each photo. Keep one set in your wallet and another tacked onto the refrigerator. These pictures form the foundation of your motivation.

You'll also need to take an accurate measurement of your waistline. All you need is an inexpensive cloth tape measure. Simply measure your abdominal girth, or waist circumference. To correctly measure your waist, stand and place a tape measure around your middle. And I don't mean the "low waist," where most men wear their pants, but rather the "high waist"—at your belly button, where you are the largest. Take a deep breath and then push all of the air out of your lungs. Measure your waist before you take the next breath in.

If your waist circumference is 40 inches or greater your risk for all of the life-threatening diseases we talked about in Chapter 1, or experiencing dementia, increases dramatically. My guess is that if you are reading this book you have at least five inches to lose, and you are not alone. According to the U.S. Centers for Disease Control, the average waist circumference for American men has now reached 39.7 inches. This means that most men in America are at high risk for metabolic syndrome and all the adverse consequences.

A second way to determine the severity of your visceral fat is by taking your waist and hip measurements to determine your index of central obesity. Known as waist-to-hip ratio (WHR), this is calculated by dividing your waist circumference by your hip circumference. Use the number from the exercise above to determine your waist measurement. The hip measurement is taken at the largest circumference around the buttocks. If your WHR is greater than 0.9 you are considered to be clinically obese.

Another measure of central obesity is the waist-to-height ratio, abbreviated as WHtR. This is determined by taking your waist circumference and dividing it by your height. For men of all ages, maintaining a WHtR of 0.5 is critical. In other words, your waist circumference should be no more than half of your height. Some doctors may tell you that as you get older, this number can shift to 0.6, but I don't agree. We have to stop thinking that it's acceptable to get fatter as we get older. Doctors used to believe that it was okay for your blood pressure to increase as you got older, but now we know that's not the case. Today, we strive to keep blood pressure in a perfect range no matter what your age, and we need to do the same with our weight and waist measurements.

Measuring Percentage Body Fat

Measuring body fat is more difficult and less accurate. The most common tool used to determine body fat percentage is a skinfold caliper, which measures skinfold thickness in millimeters and is converted in a complex equation into body fat percentage. Calipers do not measure visceral fat, they measure only subcutaneous fat. The best way to measure visceral fat at home is by measuring your waist and comparing your results each week.

You can buy your own calipers or get tested at your local gym. However, the results are only as good as the tester. The test requires someone else to determine the thickness of skinfolds at various sites on your body, including the back of your upper arm (triceps), front of the upper arm (biceps), back below the shoulder blades (subscapular), and waist. The measurements are then plugged into an equation to determine your body fat percentage. But there are more than 100 different calculations to choose from. Ensure that your tester is using the most accurate equation, or you may come up with a result that is completely misleading.

However, for the purposes of this program, you can also use the skinfold caliper to check your progress without the difficult equations. The best place to measure is just to the side of your belly button. Pick a spot and always measure at the same place in order to really follow your fat loss.

The next level of testing involves charting your measurements against population averages. Most healthcare professionals rely on a formula called the body mass index (BMI), which takes into account your current weight and height to determine whether you are overweight. This index is calculated by multiplying your weight by 705, dividing the result by your height in inches, and then dividing again by your height in inches. If your BMI is between 25 and 30 you are considered heavy, and if it is greater than 30 you're obese. The BMI range you should be shooting for is between 18 and 25.

This simplified approach works fairly well when we look at large populations of people, but because it takes into account only weight and height, it misses fatness. Every man who is muscular is considered overweight according to the BMI, even if they are lean—because of their increased muscle weight. At the same time, there are plenty of men who have a great BMI but have way too much abdominal fat and very little muscle mass. This is particularly common with older men who have lost muscle mass from lack of exercise. This condition is called normal weight obese syndrome.

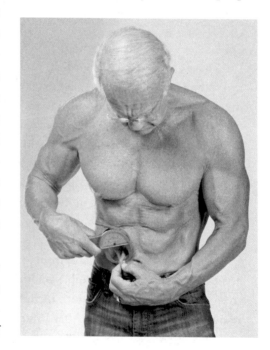

Many people confuse BMI with body fat percentage. These two things are not the same. Body fat percentage, when taken accurately, helps form a much clearer picture of health and disease risk, especially when such factors as location of body fat—such as belly fat—are taken into consideration. Body fat percentage sheds light on body fat composition where BMI cannot, which is why this calculation is often misleading.

The absolute best test we have for measuring body fat is the Dual-Energy X-ray Absorptiometry (DEXA) scan. This is a safe, X-ray device that is used primarily to determine bone mineral density, and it also does an excellent job measuring total body composition. Many doctors like me can perform one right in their office. When you have your body composition test, you keep your clothing on, and the test takes about 25 minutes and is pain-free. Once your test is complete, you will receive results outlining your percentage of body fat, fat mass, lean muscle mass, and bone density. These numbers can also help you set goals for muscle building once you're ready to enter a full exercise program like the ones outlined in *The Life Plan* or *Mastering the Life Plan*. Once you find a doctor who can perform a DEXA scan, make sure that the machine is calibrated to identify body composition.

REAL MEN, REAL MOTIVATION: LETTERS FROM MY PATIENTS

Dr. Life,

I have experienced extraordinary results since you became my doctor four years ago. While I am fortunate to have excellent health, I had never been able to achieve my goal of gaining a significant amount of lean muscle mass. It was not that I hadn't tried. I began progressive resistance training about 30 years ago. During the 1980s I trained at the World Gym in Santa Monica, California. I became a personal friend of Joe Gold and many of the most famous bodybuilders in the world at that time. Arnold Schwarzenegger, Tom Platz, Mike Mentzer, and many other famous names in the bodybuilding world trained in the Venice and Santa Monica area. Arnold taught me how to train abdominals, Tom Platz gave me tips on training legs, and Mike Mentzer gave me advice on training arms.

Even though I trained hard, from the early 1980s up to about four years ago I was never able to gain any respectable amount of lean muscle mass. When I met you I was given several physical evaluations including a DEXA scan to determine my precise amount of lean muscle mass. After I started the program I noticed my body began changing and I started gaining lean muscle mass at a steady rate. The most recent DEXA scan indicates I have gained 22 pounds of lean muscle mass on your program.

My grandson recently became a father, which makes me a great-grandfather. To put things in the right perspective, I have made dramatically more progress on your program in just four years as a grandfather and great-grandfather than I did in over 25 years, including the years I was a young man.

Jay S.

Your "Before" Numbers

You'll start your fat-loss program by memorizing your current weight and body fat percentage. Then, check in with these same measurements at least once every two weeks, at the end of one of the Life Plan Diet Cycles. And don't forget to take your starting front and side photos and repeat these photos monthly.

Starting Date:	Week 2	Week 4	Week 6	Week 8
Current Weight:				
Waist Circumference:				
WHR:				
WHtR:				
Skinfold Caliper Measurements:				
■ Triceps:				
■ Biceps:				
■ Subscapular:				
■ Waist:				
BMI:				
DEXA Results:				
■ Bone Density:				
■ Percentage of Body Fat:				
■ Fat Mass:				
■ Lean Muscle Mass:				

How Much Should You Lose?

The typical fad diets are all about dropping weight fast, yet the end result, for men in particular, is not so appealing. When men lose weight quickly they will drop both fat and muscle. So even though they lost weight, these men look like smaller, shrunken versions of the way they were before they started the diet. Then they celebrate their success by going back to their old ways, and slowly but surely they gain back the lost body fat. The killer is that their muscle mass doesn't return. If you continue to repeat this approach you'll end up becoming a fat, frail man.

I want something better for you, and that is to get both leaner and stronger. The high protein and moderate caloric restriction allow you to lose weight but to do so slowly, and without jeopardizing your muscle mass and strength. The biggest drop in weight will come at the beginning of the diet. After a few weeks, your weight loss will slow down until you begin a vigorous exercise program, which will then allow you to lose even more body fat at a faster rate. The good news is that you will lower your percent body fat by following my diet; the bad news is that the lower it gets, the slower your fat loss becomes.

During the first eight weeks of the diet you will lose weight, and your success will be visible on the scale. But once you start a full-on exercise program, your muscle mass will increase and then the numbers on the scale will begin to rise. That's why you can't worry about getting down to a specific weight as your ultimate goal. It's much more important to focus on how your pants feel and what your weekly waist measurements are showing.

Your goal is to get your percent body fat low enough so that you can see your abdominal muscles, at least first thing in the morning. Every guy's dream is to have a toned abdomen with muscle definition: a washboard stomach, a six-pack. This is not an unreasonable goal, and it will affect not only the way you look now, but your longevity as well. When you get your body fat percentage way down, to 12 percent or under, and you can see your abs, you'll also reduce your risk factors for vascular disease.

When I'm really lean, down around 7 to 8 percent body fat, I will have a six-pack all day. But if I have 10 to 12 percent body fat and the day continues normally, my six-pack starts to disappear around lunchtime. When you get up in the morning, your visceral fat cells are not swollen. But as you go about your day and you eat and start accumulating fluid in your visceral fat cells, your belly gets bigger. When the content of your abdominal cavity increases, it causes your stomach to stick out, and it eliminates the six-pack.

The average man can get that, but it takes hard work and a real commitment. For me, that means I cannot deviate from my exercise program, mostly the cardio part, and I have to focus on clean eating and not drinking alcohol. Any guy can do this. But the question is, will he? I will tell you that the health and self-esteem rewards are phenomenal for those who pull this off.

Start Thinking Like a Lean, Fit Man

The three most important components of any weight-loss program are calorie restriction, exercise, and behavioral therapy. Don't let anyone tell you differently: You cannot lose weight if you don't burn more calories than you consume in conjunction with making permanent lifestyle changes so that you can maintain your weight loss forever. The rest of the book will show you how you're going to accomplish a daily caloric deficit by eating cleaner and burning more calories through exercise. But what separates this diet from all others is getting you to change the way you think about food, and yourself, right now.

I'm not going to lie: Dieting can be difficult. But there are ways that you can make it easier for yourself so that you don't fall back into your old eating habits. For me, a big part of what keeps me going is my mindset. I look at eating as just another part of my workout: It's what I know I have to do for my body in order to look good and feel great. That's why my diet is so rigid. I know that if I follow it exactly I will be able to lose weight when I need to, and maintain my weight the rest of the time. I've left very little room for error on this plan, and I think that this structure is the key to my success.

Because I know that science supports this diet, I also know that there's only one thing holding you back from losing weight, and that's you. Anyone can eat less than he did yesterday, and most men can exercise (once they get the go-ahead from their doctor). However, my secret has always been that from the first day I decided to lose weight I shifted my thinking, creating my own behavioral therapy program. Instead of feeling sorry for myself that I was out of shape and fat, I started thinking like a lean, fit man. My self-talk, the inner monologue that runs through my head to this day, helps me continue to make good food decisions and is the first voice I hear when I make bad ones.

I tell myself the following lessons with both persistence and consistency. And when I make mistakes or bad food choices, I don't use these lessons to beat myself up. Instead,

I focus on all the things I've accomplished and how much better I feel than when I was heavy and unhealthy.

In the mornings, I remind myself of the following:

- Today I'm taking care of my health.

- Today I'll choose foods that will help prevent my having a heart attack.

- Today I'll choose foods that will help me avoid diabetes, cancer, and Alzheimer's disease.

- Today I'll choose foods that support my ability to exercise effectively.

- Today I'll choose foods that will increase my hormone levels naturally.

- Today I'll choose foods that will slow aging down and help me not get old.

Then, throughout the day, I remember the following lessons, especially before I eat.

Everything I put in my mouth can either heal me or kill me. One of the first shifts that I made in my thinking was the realization that I had to start eating for my health instead of eating for pleasure. Even when I'm dining with friends or taking my wife, Annie, out for a special dinner, I'm eating strategically. Whether I'm eating at home or eating out, I choose meals that are on the Life Plan Diets so that I don't sabotage my chances for success. I don't feel deprived when I have to pass on dessert or even some of my old favorites, because I know that the pleasure I'd get from eating them today is nothing compared to the years of better health I've been able to have, and, I hope, will continue to have, by forgoing them. In this way I'm practicing delayed gratification: I'd much rather watch my body's composition improve, see the fat melt away, and watch my muscle mass and strength increase than have the instant pleasure from eating something that's unhealthy.

This doesn't mean that I'm not enjoying what I'm eating. Some people believe that eating for health means that everything about diet foods will taste terrible. Not so! Once you switch gears and start thinking about long-term gains rather than short-term rewards, healthy foods will begin to taste better, and you will begin to enjoy and look forward to eating healthfully at every meal.

Don't give in to cravings. A craving is your brain's way of telling you it's time to eat. It is not a command to overindulge. When a craving begins, determine how you want to deal with it. It is truly up to you. Remember, a craving is similar to a wave in the ocean. It grows in intensity, peaks, and then subsides if you do not give in. Picture yourself as a surfer who is trying to "ride the wave," instead of being wiped out by it. The more you practice riding the wave, the easier it will become.

When you start to follow the Life Plan Diet, you'll find that your cravings for bad foods will go away within one to two weeks. During this transition time you'll need to prepare for these cravings so that you'll know what to do when they come on strong.

Start by having a clear vision of what you want to look like and how you want to feel, and let that guide your food choices. Your goals should be the central thing you think about, not the foods that you aren't eating. Visualize how you are benefiting from eating healthy foods. Every Life Plan meal should be eaten with awareness of how your body responds to it. Imagine the nutrients entering your bloodstream and making your muscles bigger and stronger. Healthy, fiber-rich foods are reversing plaque and improving the elasticity of your blood vessels, flowing into each and every muscle fiber and organ and making you healthier.

Before you go ahead and eat something bad, imagine exactly what that food is going to do to your body and your mind. I visualize what will happen when the blood flowing through my arteries on its way to my heart and brain suddenly stops when a big clot forms at a site of inflammation caused by the food or drink I was thinking of putting into my mouth. Sugary foods and drinks will turn me into an old man, or worse, a dead man. This really works for me: Just thinking about the damage these foods will cause really gets me past my cravings.

Sometimes, when I start thinking about foods and drinks that I really want that are bad for me, such as chocolate, cookies, French fries, or vodka, I look at my "before" photo, and before I know it, the craving is gone. Once you start carrying around your "before" photos, and remember to look at them, you'll be able to beat your cravings, too. Best of all, you'll know that you have control over food, instead of food controlling you. Defuse your cravings when you feel them coming on by remembering my "3 Ds."

- DELAY eating anything for at least 10 minutes so that your action is conscious, not impulsive.

- DISTRACT yourself by engaging in an activity that requires concentration, including exercise.

- DISTANCE yourself from the food: Get up and go where the food you want is not available.

Healthy foods are your friends, not your enemies. Eating healthfully is not a punishment, it's a gift. A lot of men view eating healthy as something they have to do but don't like. However, if you look at these choices in a very positive way, recalling that they're going to help you build muscle, get rid of body fat, clean up your arteries, and help you live a longer, healthier life, it changes your attitude about these foods.

The real enemies are the foods you know you have to avoid, even if they've been providing you comfort in the past. These foods are the high-glycemic carbohydrates, sweets, or fried foods. You'll also have to pass on the beverages that pretend to be your friend, such as alcohol, carbonated soft drinks, and so-called healthy fruit juices.

View hunger as a good thing. We've been told by our society to view hunger as a negative experience. View hunger as a good thing. If you're truly hungry you know you're in a caloric deficit, and what you are feeling is your body tapping into its fat stores. Then, instead of rushing off to eat something in order to get rid of the hunger pangs, you can hold off a little and stretch out the time in between meals so you can burn more fat. You'll also be better able to discriminate between hunger, boredom, and cravings if you can delay eating.

Some men can deal with a little bit of hunger, but they can't deal with a lot of hunger. Others get irritable when they don't eat. The best way I've found to deal with making sure that I don't become irritable is to eat small meals throughout the day. You need to start your day with a healthy breakfast (this doesn't mean a huge breakfast), then eat every three hours. On this diet you'll learn how to eat more often, instead of less, with the goal being four, or five, or even six small meals a day with protein as part of each meal. If you eat every three hours you're not going to get hungry, your body will not be pushing you to eat something you shouldn't, and you will have better control over your cravings.

Focus on your future weight, not your present weight. Many men get up in the morning and weigh themselves, then become agitated when they don't see a big dip in the numbers, and in disgust eat an enormous breakfast and continue to binge throughout the day. Lean, fit men don't get on the scale very often, so I discourage this when you first start the program. Instead, focus on your belly, on how your pants feel, and less on what the scale says. Keep your eyes on the prize, as they say, and weigh yourself only when you notice a big change in how you look or feel.

Surround yourself with role models. Choose to spend your time with people you really admire who have become fit and lean, and listen to what they say. My first fitness role model back in 1998 was Porter Freeman. He was the first winner in my age group of the Body-*for*-LIFE contest. When his pictures came out, I realized that he was about 10 years younger than I was, and his before picture looked just about as bad as I did. Now he looked terrific. I saw his pictures and read his story, and quickly I related to his experiences and realized that if a former bartender could actually stop drinking and follow a really rigid diet, train hard, and change himself, I should be able to do it as well. I kept thinking about Porter as I trained for the contest, and he really motivated my success.

Lean, fit people will also have a positive subconscious effect on your success. A 2007 Harvard Medical School study showed that your weight will basically balance toward the people you spend time with. Researchers found that a person's chances of becoming obese increased by 57 percent if he or she had a friend who became obese, and similar findings occurred among pairs of adult siblings. Persons of the same sex had relatively greater influence on each other than those of the opposite sex. So while obesity is not contagious, the study shows that we are predisposed to adopt the habits of others; so why not adopt good habits rather than poor ones?

Last, build a support team to help you succeed. Your team could include your family, your work associates, or even the guys at the gym. Your role as part of the team is to share your successes. Once a week, show off your new abdominal measurements and photos and talk about how much further you have to go to achieve your goals.

Set a good example for your family. As odd as it seems, our children are predicted to have a shorter life span than their parents, according to Dr. David S. Ludwig, director of the obesity program at Children's Hospital Boston, because of the prevalence and severity of obesity and its associated diseases and complications. This is the first time in human history that this has ever happened. We need to set a better example for our children and grandchildren. If a father or a grandfather is really fit, his kids and his grandkids will take notice, and they'll start trying to find out what he's doing differently than everyone else. Be a responsible husband, partner, father, and grandfather. Your family needs you and wants you more than you realize. Even when you think that everyone in your family is ignoring you, they will be very disappointed if you don't live to your full potential, because you matter to them. And you'll also see that even when they tease you about your newfound eating habits as you follow this diet, you are both consciously and unconsciously motivating them to make positive changes in their own lives.

Think of dieting as fun, not drudgery. There's no way to hide the fact that dieting is a challenge. But viewing the process as a contest instead of a chore makes all the difference in my mindset. Men love a challenge, so use this warrior mentality to your advantage. Whenever I need to lose a few pounds—for a photo shoot or when I find myself way off track—I create mini goals, and when I meet them, I set slightly higher goals to achieve. Sometimes, I treat myself to a massage in order to reinforce how good I feel about the weight I lost. I test the limits of my hunger (more on that later) and I revel in my success.

One of my favorite rewards is to sneak on a pair of my slimmest pants. Recently I had a couple of pairs of pants that I wanted to wear, but I couldn't. My goal was to be able to wear those pants. Then, once a week I put them on until they fit. I also keep my fat pants. Every now and then, I put them on to reinforce what I've accomplished, and it just keeps me on track. If you find yourself getting off track, that's when you get out your old pants and put them on to remind you that if you don't get back on track, you'll end up filling up those pants again.

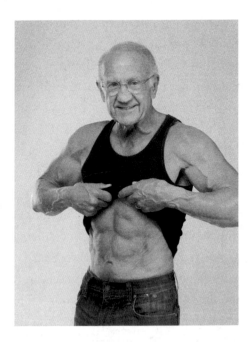

Get organized to get thin. The better I can organize my life, the easier it is to stay on my program. I think mental organization is a real important feat for anyone who wants to achieve healthy goals. When your mind is cluttered with a bunch of stuff, it's really hard to focus on what you need to do to really get healthy, and fit, and lean.

One way to get better organized is to learn to rely on yourself. You need to start taking personal responsibility for your health. You can do this by becoming an expert in health and fitness (and of course, you're taking the first step just by reading my book). I've found that the fittest men I know are always looking for new ways to improve their workouts, or searching out new recipes or healthy alternatives. Check out my website (www.drlife.com) for information about health and fitness.

Another way to stay organized is to think of this program not as a diet, but as a long-term lifestyle. By doing so, you'll be better able to follow it consistently. If you follow these plans every single meal of every single day of every week with the exception of one meal, you'll quickly see that you can make conscious and organized decisions.

With the right mindset, great things can happen. Let's get moving toward making the second half of your life the best half.

CHAPTER 4

The Science Supporting the Life Plan Diet

The foods you eat and drink every day become the deal breakers or the deal makers in terms of having a lean, fit, healthy body. You can have perfectly balanced hormones, and you can religiously follow a perfect daily workout, but if you don't eat right you will not get lean. You will not become fit. You will not improve your health. Diet is the key to a successful program of fitness, leanness, and great health.

The premise of the Life Plan Diet is not to simply adopt the mantra "eat less and exercise more." I'll leave that one to the many fad diets out there. If you're reading this book, you've probably tried some of those, and may even have achieved good results at first. However, fad diets that severely restrict calories or food choices form the foundation of a practice that is ultimately unsustainable, and so is the weight loss. Eventually, the pounds creep back, and your waistline becomes bigger than ever.

In order to achieve the most efficient and lasting fat loss we need to get off the roller coaster of fad diets and instead train your body to affect the primary mechanism necessary for burning body fat: your metabolism. This is the ability to use and burn the calories that you take in from the foods you eat instead of storing those calories as body fat. Increasing your metabolism is what allows you to create a true caloric deficit and at the same time provide you with the energy you'll need once you are ready to follow a full exercise program. The best part is that a diet that boosts your metabolic rate will almost instantly make you feel more alive and awake, because when you use and burn food more efficiently, you are creating more energy. If you generally feel sluggish during the day you'll notice a very significant change once you start following the program.

Our metabolic rate is partially determined by our genetics, but is also affected by our activity level, diet, overall health, and body fat composition. The healthier and more active we are, the faster our metabolic rates become and the better we are at burning body fat. Muscle tissue at rest burns far more calories than the same amount of body fat: The more muscle you have, the more calories you can burn throughout the day. At the same time, your body fat requires very few calories to sustain itself. That means you don't have to continue to overeat to maintain body fat, whereas muscle requires many more calories to sustain its mass and metabolic functions.

And contrary to popular belief, your age has very little effect on your metabolic rate. As people age many believe they need to physically slow down, so they do just that. They use their age as an excuse not to move around, so their metabolic rate does indeed decline. But those who develop the attitude that to avoid getting old they must continue moving and keeping their metabolic rate at high levels thrive and enjoy a youthful life.

While we can't change our genetics, we can control the other factors that influence metabolism. The first step is to boost metabolism by swapping out bad food choices for good ones that will increase muscle mass and require more calories for the body to process. The foods on the Life Plan Diet are chosen specifically for their ability to increase metabolism. My program is based on the concept of *Diet-Induced Thermogenesis* (DIT). DIT involves knowing how many calories the body uses to digest, metabolize, and store the foods we eat. We know that it takes more energy to digest and convert proteins and complex carbohydrates than it does for fats and sugars. This is why I focus on small, frequent meals that are high in protein and complex carbs, which will burn more efficiently and leave fewer calories for storage. Foods that have a low DIT include all processed foods that are high in carbohydrates and fat and are the foods we must completely avoid: white bread, white rice, French fries, cheese, and alcohol—in other words, most of the trigger foods we've talked about earlier. The foods we will focus on are the highest-DIT foods, which include:

- Chicken

- Turkey

- Lean red meats

- Peanut butter

- Brown rice

- Wild rice

- Yams

- Green vegetables

- Apples

- Nontropical fruits

High-DIT meals burn more calories than meals with low DITs even when they have the same number of calories. This is why simply counting calories never works in the long run. For example, a plain peanut butter sandwich on whole grain bread may have the same number of calories as a ham sandwich with mayonnaise on white bread. However, the peanut butter sandwich is better for you because it has a higher DIT. Each of the meals on the Life Plan Diet is designed to maximize its DIT.

DIT calories are burned without our having to do any exercise, because we have to eat and digest our food in order to survive. By choosing the right foods you can begin to lose weight without even trying. Ultimately, when you combine exercise with a high-DIT diet, the pounds will fly off, because both cardio and resistance training exercise boosts metabolism.

When you follow a DIT plan, there really is a best time to eat to maximize the DIT. A 1993 study published in the *American Journal of Clinical Nutrition* researched the relationship between DIT and the time meals were eaten. These scientists were able to demonstrate that if a meal is eaten in the morning, 16 percent of its calories are used to metabolize the meal. When the same meal is eaten in the afternoon, 13.5 percent of its calories are needed to metabolize the food. When the meal is eaten at night, only 10.9 percent of its calories are used to metabolize the food. The meal you eat in the morning gets the most thermogenic response. At night, you are allowing foods with high-DIT calories to be stored as body fat rather than being used by your body to process the food. The problem here is that most men consume the largest proportion of their calories in the evening.

On the Life Plan Diet you will consume the majority of your calories by 6:00 or 7:00 p.m. If you must eat after that, choose lean proteins (a small piece of chicken, or a tablespoon or two of natural, no-sugar-added peanut butter) and avoid fats and carbohydrates. Only 3 percent of fat calories are used for DIT, while 23 percent of carbohydrate calories and a whopping 30 percent of protein calories are burned as a result of DIT. That means if you stick with proteins as a late-night snack, you'll burn off most of it.

This research is just one more reason why breakfast still is the most important meal of the day. Yet every overfat/obese man I have ever met has told me he doesn't eat breakfast. Skipping meals—especially breakfast—in order to limit calories is the number-one reason for failing to achieve lifelong leanness and muscularity. It is also the main cause of eating the wrong foods later in the day. Every time you miss a meal your blood sugar drops, increasing your hunger and cravings. This leads at the very least to overeating later in the day, or at the very worst making terrible food choices to eat what's easy and available, rather than what's good for you. Poor control invariably means you will eat foods that are high in calories and low in nutrients; the very thing you are trying to avoid.

The Right Nutrients Make All the Difference

Other foods on the Life Plan Diet increase metabolism in a different way: by supplying your body with the nutrients it needs. While there are zillions of different kinds of foods, there are really only three types of nutrients you need to worry about: protein, carbohydrates, and fats. Every type of food falls into one of these categories.

I have a simple rule that will help you balance each meal and that's easy to remember. Each meal will consist of:

- 1 part fat

- 2 parts protein

- 3 parts healthy carbohydrates

The Power of Protein

Because of the amino acids they contain, foods high in protein are the building blocks of muscle and are an essential part of the human diet for the growth and repair of tissue. Adequate protein is necessary for optimizing hormones, increasing lean body mass, and decreasing body fat. Eating foods high in protein is the single most important way you can improve vascular health, because they form the basis of a noninflammatory diet.

We also know that proteins, by far, require the most calories to burn. It takes roughly 30 percent of the calories that we burn every day just to digest food. Protein digestion alone requires about a third of those calories. That means the more protein you eat, the more calories your body is using to transfer food to energy. In other words, just eating meals that are high in protein increases the number of calories that you burn as a result of digestion by as much as 33 percent. If you incorporate protein in every meal, you can really maximize the surge effect of using calories to metabolize the food you're eating. This is totally effortless weight loss: You are literally sitting around doing nothing but burning calories. When you follow an eating program like the one I'm talking about that is high in essential amino acids, you're going to naturally start whittling away at your body fat, especially when your carbohydrate intake is low.

Finally, protein is essential to maintaining and increasing testosterone and growth hormone production. The best diet to achieve optimal sexual function and optimal sexual health is one that contains the most amino acids. Examples of quality proteins are:

- Beans

- Chicken or turkey

- Eggs

- Fish

- Lean meats

- Low-fat cottage cheese

- Low-fat yogurt

- Protein shakes

- Soy products (soybeans, tofu, tempeh)

The meal plans on this diet provide about 180 grams of protein per day, which falls right in the recommended range for muscle and strength building. If you've read other diet books, you may notice that this is much higher than most nutritionists will recommend. I choose high levels because your goal should be preparing your body for regular, vigorous exercise, and you'll need this much protein to support your workouts. On this diet you'll be eating 20 to 30 grams of protein per meal. Each serving should be about the size and thickness of your palm. Consuming more than that is not more beneficial; in fact, it's problematic. Excess protein beyond one gram per pound of body weight is often simply excreted or stored as body fat, which doesn't help if you're trying to get leaner.

Some doctors used to say that eating too much protein would negatively affect your kidney function. That's something I've heard throughout my medical career. However, that statement applies only to people who are already having some kidney dysfunction. While it's true that people who have some kidney failure should not be eating high-protein diets, I have never, and I mean never, encountered anybody who has gotten into trouble eating a high-protein diet. It is a myth, and it's a myth that was debunked: It's just not a problem.

The quality of your protein choices is more important than whether they are organic or not. However, in all respects, organic meats that are grass-fed are the best choice. Organic refers to the lack of chemicals used in the growing of a plant or raising of an animal. Free-range animal meats contain a better ratio of good to bad fats compared to traditionally raised animals that are fed grains to fatten them up faster. Grass contains omega-3 fatty acids, which have anti-inflammatory effects, whereas grains contain more omega-6 fatty acids, which have a pro-inflammatory effect. Nonorganic meats contain certain amounts of antibiotics and bovine growth hormone. Hormone-free animal and dairy products are recommended in my diet.

How the Body Reacts to Protein

These are the signals your body is sending about your current protein consumption:

- If you are usually hungry 1 to 2 hours after a meal you are not eating enough protein.

- If you are hungry 3 to 4 hours after a meal your protein intake is optimal.

- If you are not hungry for 5 to 7 hours after a meal you ate too much protein during your last meal.

The Right Fats Keep You Feeling Satisfied

Healthy types of dietary fat allow your body to feel satisfied after eating, build hormones, insulate and protect your organs, and transport nutrients throughout your body. Eating fat is not problematic; eating the wrong *types* of fat is, because too much of the wrong kinds of fats can contribute to premature aging. It is therefore very important for you to have some basic knowledge about the difference between healthy fats and unhealthy fats so that you can make intelligent decisions.

Assessing the many types and forms of dietary fat can seem complicated, but ultimately the bottom line is: The optimal types of fat are found in natural foods, such as fish, nuts, seeds, olives, and animal proteins. Dietary fats found in processed foods are *not* healthy.

Trans Fats/Hydrogenated Fats

By far the worst fat options are hydrogenated (or partially hydrogenated) fats, which are liquid oils that have been artificially saturated with hydrogen atoms to create a solid fat with a longer shelf life. Margarine and vegetable shortening are examples of this highly unnatural type of fat. Hydrogenated and partially hydrogenated fats also contain trans-fatty acids, a type of fatty acid that is not created in the body and is rarely found in nature. Trans-fatty acids (otherwise known as trans fats) are found in fried foods. They increase serum levels of "bad" cholesterol (LDL—remember "L" equals lethal) and decrease the "good" cholesterol (HDL—remember "H" equals healthy) and are heavily associated with coronary heart disease. They have been shown to adversely affect metabolic processes in heart tissue. Trans fats are also incorporated into cell membranes even though they are not normal components of human tissue. When this occurs they interfere with the function of cell membranes, making your cells less flexible and blocking natural biochemical pathways. Worst of all, researchers at Wake Forest University found that trans fats increase the amount of belly fat and redistribute fat tissue to the abdomen from other parts of the body.

Hydrogenated and partially hydrogenated oils were used extensively in commercially prepared foods, including peanut butter, mayonnaise, baked goods, margarine, and chocolate. In recent years public awareness about trans fats has put pressure on food manufacturers, and many shy away from using them. Of this list, the only food allowed on the Life Plan Diet is peanut butter, so it will be easy to avoid exposure to trans fats from these other sources. When you buy peanut butter, read the ingredients label carefully, and purchase one whose *only* ingredient is peanuts.

Saturated Fats

Saturated fats are solid at room temperature. Butter, cheese, and cream are all high in saturated fat, as is the fat in meat and tropical oils (coconut, palm, and palm kernel oil). Saturated fats increase the amount of "bad" cholesterol (LDL) in the blood, which can lead to heart disease. When saturated fats are incorporated into your cell membranes the membranes tend to become rigid and less flexible, which in turn can affect their receptor mechanisms. This may explain why saturated fats are associated with insulin resistance and type 2 diabetes. In addition, diets high in animal fat are associated with colon cancer. All of these adverse effects can be avoided simply by replacing saturated fats with "healthy fats"—monounsaturated fats.

Monounsaturated Fats

Monounsaturated fats are usually liquid at room temperature but may solidify in the refrigerator. Monounsaturated oils include olive oil, peanut oil, avocado oil, and canola oil. These oils have no effect on insulin levels. Because they aren't harmful they can be considered healthful. Long-term consumption of these oils (especially olive oil) in several southern European countries is associated with low overall mortality rates and low incidence of coronary heart disease. For cooking, your best choice is olive oil—preferably cold-pressed and unrefined ("extra-virgin")—over both butter and margarine.

Polyunsaturated Fats

Safflower, sunflower, corn, sesame, and soy all contain polyunsaturated fatty acids (PUFAs). Even though they are cholesterol-free and low in saturated fat, overexposure to oils from these plants can still cause problems by creating free radicals that damage DNA, alter cell membranes, and promote cancer.

Safflower oil is the most unsaturated vegetable oil, and as such can cause significant immune suppression. This is surprising news to many consumers who were told that polyunsaturated oils were part of a healthy diet.

Essential Fatty Acids

Omega-3 and omega-6 fatty acids are both essential fatty acids that the body cannot make. The "essential" part refers to the fact that we need these fats to promote a healthy diet. A deficiency in them is detrimental to our physical and mental well-being, causing serious diseases, including stroke, heart disease, rheumatoid and degenerative arthritis, skin problems including wrinkles, loss of vision, and degenerative brain diseases. Many men (especially those who are currently following a low-fat diet) suffer from an essential fatty acid deficiency. Therefore, we must make sure we eat foods that contain them.

There are three main types of omega-3 fats—EPA (eicosapentaenoic acid), DHA (docosahexaenoic acid), and ALA (alpha-linolenic acid). EPA and DHA are the "marine" omega-3s found in fish; ALA is found mostly in plant oils. Most authorities believe that EPA and DHA are the omega-3 fats that play the greatest role in promoting health and preventing disease. ALA (found in flaxseed) is an indirect source of EPA and DHA. However, we can convert only less than 15 percent of ALA into EPA and DHA, so most experts think flaxseed is a poor way to get adequate amounts of EPA and DHA.

Unfortunately, omega-3 fatty acids are not nearly as plentiful in the foods we eat today, because food companies have deliberately destroyed them in order to increase the shelf life of their products. Meat from today's cows and chickens has much less omega-3 fatty acids, since these animals are fed processed grains that are low in omega-3s instead of wild plants and seeds, which are naturally high in these fats. As a result, we now consume one-sixth the amount of omega-3 fatty acids that our ancestors did.

The Life Plan Diet can be high in omega-3s when you avoid foods fried in vegetable oils such as corn and safflower and eliminate processed foods. At the same time you will increase the amount of omega-3s in your diet by eating green leafy vegetables and more oily fish. For those who don't like fish, fish oil supplements are now an option: You should take three to four grams per day. Cooking with canola oil instead of vegetable oil also helps, as well as choosing foods that are fortified with omega-3s, including certain types of eggs. Omega-3 eggs are laid by chickens that have been fed flaxseeds.

The best choice for increasing omega-3s is fish. And of all fish, the ones to choose include the following. Feel free to swap any of these for the fish suggestions on my diet, as long as you keep the quantities the same:

- Bluefish

- Flounder

- Herring

- Mackerel

- Salmon

- Sardines

- Shrimp

- Swordfish

The Craziness Surrounding Carbs

Thirty years ago the American Heart Association advertised that high-carbohydrate/low-fat diets were the only way to eat in order to avoid heart disease and achieve ultimate health. This advice gave many of us full license to eat any and all carbs with little or no regard to whether they were healthy choices. The profit-motivated food manufacturers jumped on the bandwagon and hooked us all on fast food, cheap pasta dinners, processed baked goods, and low-fat, more expensive dairy products.

How wrong they were! We now know that there are all kinds of carbohydrates, and that some choices are definitely better for us than others. We do need carbohydrates in our diet, but they need to be the right carbohydrates—carbohydrates that don't spike blood sugars and insulin levels.

Man-made carbohydrates come from grains. All of these undergo processing that removes most of their natural fiber and nutrients, making them easily digestible so that they are rapidly assimilated by our bodies. These carbohydrates have very high glycemic indexes (a measure of how fast a particular food will raise your blood sugar that you'll read more about below), and they literally mainline sugar into the bloodstream, pushing blood sugars and insulin levels sky-high. When they are fully digested, blood sugar levels fall, hunger returns, and cravings and compulsive, uncontrolled eating take over. This vicious cycle is replayed day in and day out throughout America by those who have bought into the high-carb/low-fat mindset.

Vegetables and most fruits are healthy carbohydrates, because they are full of fiber and antioxidants. They are digested very slowly and enter the bloodstream in small amounts, which gently and gradually increase blood sugar levels.

The goal of any good diet is never to reduce all carbohydrates, just the ones that are easily converted into simple sugars. Sugar is toxic; it's just that simple. Many experts are now considering the campaign against sugar to be as important as the war on tobacco.

By eliminating as much sugar from your diet as possible you'll be able take more control of your health and stop cravings once and for all. But sugar has become an insidious part of our daily diet. Without knowing it, you may be eating an average of 20 teaspoons of sugar every day. That's 320 calories daily, or 117,000 calories a year, which our bodies convert into 33 pounds of body fat. This doesn't include the natural sugars found in fruits vegetables and milk—it's just the sugar that the food manufactures add to our foods.

Beyond the obvious (white, raw, brown, or cane sugar; corn syrup or high-fructose corn syrup; molasses, maple syrup, honey, or sorghum syrup; fruit juice concentrate, jams and jellies, sugary drinks, and desserts), sugar can be found in just about every processed food you can imagine, from yogurt and sauces to bread and peanut butter. Unknowingly, Americans now consume 130 pounds of sugar per person a year—that's a third of a pound every day. The American Heart Association recommends that men should not consume more than 150 calories of added sugar a day: That's less than the amount in just one can of soda.

New research is showing that when it comes to sugar, all calories are not created equal. The latest studies from the University of California, Davis suggest that calories from added sugars are different from calories from other foods. Researcher Kimber Stanhope found that the subjects in her study who consumed high-fructose corn syrup had increased blood levels of LDL cholesterol and other risk factors for cardiovascular disease in as little as two weeks of exposure. Doctors and scientists previously believed that plaque formation was a result of a high-fat, high-calorie diet. Instead, it looks as if it's the sugar, not the calories, that is the culprit.

My advice: Read labels very carefully and avoid packaged foods entirely. Almost all of them contain sugar or corn syrup. Stop adding sugar to your coffee or sweetening fresh fruit. I know that sugar is one of the hardest habits to break, but you'll find that in just a week or so you won't feel the urge to reach for the sugar bowl, and you'll find weight loss becomes a whole lot easier.

Understanding the Glycemic Index

The glycemic index determines how fast a particular food you consume will raise your blood sugar. Diabetics have successfully used the glycemic index to help control their blood sugars, but you can use this same information to help you lose fat and prevent cravings. The idea is that when blood sugar and insulin levels are kept low, your body is much less likely to convert sugars to body fat, and food cravings are reduced or even eliminated altogether. One more thing to consider: It's the high-glycemic carbs, including fruits, sweets, and fried fatty foods, that decrease testosterone and growth hormone production. Ultimately you have a choice: Continue eating high-glycemic foods or enjoy a better sex life and great health for years to come.

Using this index has worked very well for me and my patients, and I recommend it as a tool to help you get lean and stay lean. You can find a glycemic index list of some of the common foods we eat on my website: www.drlife.com. The evidence is overwhelming that the obesity and type 2 diabetes epidemics are a direct result of our obsession with high-glycemic carbohydrates.

Foods that have a high index (greater than 60) are the foods you must avoid. They include ice cream, white breads, all white flour products, bagels, white potatoes, bananas, raisins, potato chips, alcoholic beverages, white rice, and pastas made with white flour.

An ultra-low-glycemic-carbohydrate eating plan is the only way I know to beat carbohydrate addiction. On this plan your hunger will be well controlled and your food cravings and compulsive eating will come to a rapid stop. Low-glycemic-index foods (under 45) are the ones you're allowed to have, and they include:

- Beans/legumes (with the exception of baked beans and fava beans)

- Brown rice

- Colorful vegetables

- Grapes

- High-fiber, sugar-free cereals

- Nontropical fruits

- Nuts

- Steel-cut oatmeal

- Sugar-free dairy products

- Sugar-free peanut butter

- Whole wheat or whole grain foods

- Yams (sweet potatoes)

Managing Carbohydrate and Gluten Sensitivity

Carbohydrate sensitivity is a term that describes a volatile increase in blood sugar as a result of eating carbohydrates, especially those with a high glycemic index. People who have carbohydrate sensitivity produce excessive amounts of insulin—rapidly driving their blood sugars down. As they plummet, extreme hunger and cravings for sweets take over, and this vicious cycle is repeated throughout the day. Over time this can progress to full-blown insulin resistance, resulting in type 2 diabetes, serious blood vessel disease, hypertension, excessive weight gain, and premature death.

As many as 75 percent of overweight individuals are thought to be carbohydrate sensitive. And as you age, your sensitivity increases. I recommend that carbohydrate sensitivity be treated very much like any other addiction—that is, with abstinence, which means forgoing high-glycemic carbs and processed foods.

Gluten sensitivity is an entirely different issue. Gluten is a protein found in foods processed mostly from grains, primarily wheat. About one in 100 people in America have physical reactions to gluten, which in rare situations can be life-threatening. Gluten intolerance needs to be separated into three distinct categories: celiac disease, nonceliac gluten sensitivity, and wheat allergies. All of these categories of people need to avoid wheat products and other grains, including barley, rye, kamut, and spelt.

Some of the symptoms of gluten intolerance include abdominal distention, pain and cramping, and digestive issues (constipation and diarrhea). Some people with gluten sensitivity report other symptoms that affect their overall health as well as their thinking, including:

- Arthritis

- Attention deficit disorder (ADD)

- Depression, anxiety, and irritability

- Fatigue

- Hair loss (alopecia)

- Headaches and migraines

- Joint pain

- Peripheral neuropathy (including a tingling or sensation of swelling of toes and fingers)

The best way to determine if you are either gluten or carbohydrate sensitive is by keeping a food journal, like the one featured in Appendix A. Write down your reaction (both physically and emotionally) to the foods you eat. This will enable you to "listen" to what your body is telling you, and it won't take long before you can recognize which carbs adversely affect you.

Focus on High-Fiber Foods

Fiber is vitally important—especially if you want to lose belly fat. On average, American men consume around 10 grams to 12 grams of fiber per day, but the recommended intake is 25 grams to 50 grams—preferably around 35 grams. In a major study published in the *Journal of the American Heart Association* it was shown that a high intake of fiber reduces not only obesity but also high blood pressure and other heart disease risk factors, and many cancers. Some experts believe fiber plays a greater role in determining heart disease risk than total or saturated fat intake.

Dietary fiber does all of this by remaining in your GI tract. This provides bulk to the foods you eat, so that food stays in the stomach longer, leaving you feeling fuller and delaying hunger and cravings. Once fiber-rich foods reach your intestines, they move along at a faster rate, which slows the release of carbohydrates and cholesterol-raising fats into your bloodstream. Since these sugars are slowly absorbed rather than mainlined into your bloodstream, your blood sugar levels remain well controlled, and insulin secretion is reduced. Many experts now believe fiber's effect on blood sugar levels is the main reason for its "fat-fighting" properties and other health benefits.

The best fiber sources include natural, unprocessed foods such as fruits, vegetables, whole grains, and legumes. Eating these makes you feel full, so you eat much less without even thinking about it. This was really brought to light in a recent study from Penn State that showed how people eat about the same *weight* of food on a daily basis. In other words, it is not the total number of calories consumed that controls how much you eat; instead it's the volume or weight of the food that determines when you think you've had enough. When you eat high-fiber foods, you consume a higher volume of food with fewer calories—and you won't feel the least bit deprived.

A Paleo Program Is Not Always the Answer

Dieting trends of late have circled back to an old fad: very low-carb. Today it's packaged as a "Paleo" approach. Paleo diets instruct followers to eat like the cavemen did as hunters and gatherers and forgo all processed foods that contain grains, including all simple carbohydrates. These diets do a great job of controlling binge eating and cravings, especially for those who are carbohydrate or gluten sensitive, because the program rapidly achieves control over blood sugars and insulin levels, and thereby prevents the vicious cycle of high insulin levels followed by low blood sugar levels—the root cause of cravings.

However, the diet encourages high protein consumption based on foods with unhealthy levels of saturated fats. These include red meats, organ meat such as sweetbreads, lamb, pork, chicken liver, bacon, and dairy products. Even lean options eaten in excess will end up promoting a high-saturated-fat diet. When your high-protein sources are also high in saturated fats, your heart is going to suffer. Any man who wants to pursue a Paleo diet needs to make sure he hasn't inherited risk factors for heart disease, and that his cholesterol panel is in good shape. I've had patients who had great cholesterol panels, and when I repeated the testing after they followed a Paleo program for as little as three months, their levels had gone way up. Simply put, the Paleo approach is not a great option for men who have any predisposition to heart disease or have evidence of vascular disease.

We also do not know what the benefits of following a gluten-free diet are if you are not gluten sensitive and do not suffer from celiac disease. Approximately one in 100 Americans suffer from celiac, a condition that occurs when one or two genetic mutations cause the immune system to attack the walls of the intestine after one eats foods containing the protein gluten. Symptoms vary, but can include vomiting, chronic diarrhea, or constipation. Gluten sensitivity is different. It is described when someone who does not have celiac shows physical and often mental health improvements on a gluten-free diet, and worsens again when gluten is eaten. Many believe that nonceliac gluten sensitivity is a wide, unseen epidemic. Still others believe that anyone following a gluten-free diet will at least lose weight. However, the problem I see is that if you don't have gluten sensitivity or celiac, you are missing out on some important nutrients that are found in healthy grains. A single blood test can let you know if you have a true gluten sensitivity or intolerance. However, the gold standard for positively identifying celiac disease is an intestinal biopsy.

The Ultimate Metabolism Boost: Fasting

Perhaps the most straightforward way to lose belly fat is to not eat at all. Don't laugh: The science of extreme caloric restriction has shown it to be one of the few food-based interventions that extend life span. Researchers at the Intermountain Medical Center Heart

Institute reported in 2011 that fasting not only lowers one's risk of coronary artery disease and diabetes, but also causes significant changes in a person's blood cholesterol levels. Fasting was found to reduce cardiac risk factors, including triglycerides, weight, and blood sugar levels. Fasting allows the body to use stored fat as a source of fuel instead of glucose. This decreases the number of fat cells in the body, which lowers the likelihood of insulin resistance and diabetes.

Fasting has been proven not only to induce weight loss, but also to give your pancreas a break from producing insulin. According to Dr. Michael Mosley, author of *The Fastdiet*, during the first 24 hours of a fast your body experiences real change. First, research has shown that fasting may improve mood and protect the brain from dementia and cognitive decline. It also positively affects the body. The glucose circulating in your blood gets burned for energy, and when that's depleted, the body turns to the muscles and liver and uses glycogen, another form of glucose. When the glycogen has been completely depleted, the body turns to the fat stores, and that's when you will experience real weight loss. This process is called *ketogenesis*. When this happens, your brain is getting its energy from ketones, which are the breakdown of metabolized fat. Sometimes you can smell it: The ketone on your breath has the smell of acetone, the chemical in paint thinner and nail polish remover. When you become ketotic, you lose a lot of water weight. It's like a diuretic that stimulates your kidneys to secrete liquid.

Fasting literally shocks your system: It's like rebooting your computer after months of its running slowly. It shrinks the stomach and, surprisingly, it eliminates hunger pangs. It also facilitates true sugar withdrawal, which is especially important if you've developed a real addiction to carbohydrates. I've found that if I can fast for a couple of days I completely lose interest in sugar when I go back to eating, which is a real benefit for being able to maintain this eating plan over the long term. Unfortunately, a prolonged fast is not really sustainable, and ultimately will cause you to lose muscle mass.

If you want to get the benefits of fasting without total starvation, there are basically three options. The first is a lifestyle change to continuing extreme caloric restriction. Those who follow extreme caloric restriction eat sparingly throughout the day, focusing on nutrient-rich foods that contain very few calories (under 1,000 calories a day, which is 50 percent less than the average diet). These dieters not only lose weight, they see real and lasting changes to their overall health. They report decreases in blood pressure, better heart health, and increased overall energy. However, an extreme caloric restriction program won't work for men who are already heavily into an exercise program, or plan to ramp up into one, as I'm hoping you will be. You will just run out of steam and very likely hurt yourself if you don't consume enough calories to support your exercise program.

Another popular dieting trend right now is called a 5-2 diet. This is a modified fasting approach based on the idea of intermittent fasting: eating fewer calories, but only some of the time. On a typical 5-2 diet, you eat very few calories two days a week—for men that means around 600 calories. The rest of the week you are free to eat whatever you normally would eat. This type of diet also promotes weight loss, but I take issue with it. First, it doesn't help you set up better habits. If you continue with your bad eating habits, even if you are eating these foods only five days a week, you're not really training your body or your brain to make better choices. And continuing to eat these bad foods still puts you at risk for all the diseases we discussed in Chapter 1.

The absolute best approach is to eat a well-balanced diet all the time, and a similar number of calories each day. However, I do want you to experience the benefits of fasting, which I see as an opportunity to kick-start your fat-loss plan both mentally and physically. That's why the Life Plan Diet begins with the JumpStart Diet, which features a fairly easy 36-hour fast. During this time you need to drink plenty of liquids, but you will not eat. Afterward, you'll transition back into eating a well-balanced diet composed of the right amounts of protein, fat, and carbohydrates. This eating program continues to drive down glycogen, which allows the liver the ability to start metabolizing fat.

The biggest obstacle for men when it comes to dieting is the mental part. I have found that for myself, and my patients, even a brief fast not only gets great results, it builds confidence. When you complete this fast, you will have mastered something that 99 percent of the American population has never even attempted. If you can do this small step, you'll be able to reach any goal you set. I also know that men love a challenge. Fasting works like a game for me: I feel like I'm totally in control of my eating, and I rise to the challenge. It's also put food and eating into a new perspective. Now when I think I need to eat something, I can ask myself if I'm really hungry.

There are a handful of men out there who simply should not fast. If you have an underlying medical condition, discuss this program with your doctor. In fact, it's a good idea for every man to consult with his doctor before starting any new diet program. However, if you know that you have type 1 diabetes or are currently taking diabetic medications such as oral hypoglycemic agents or insulin, then you'll need to move right to Day 2 of the JumpStart program. If you have a true eating disorder that is being treated by a psychologist or physician, skip the fast until you are medically cleared. Once you have been given the okay by your health professional, you can go back and try the fast whenever you want.

Transitioning Back to Eating

The optimal eating pattern for maintaining blood sugar levels at an even range throughout the day is to eat five to six small meals a day that are roughly 200 to 300 calories each. When you do that, you don't get hungry. The brain doesn't sense that you're starving, and you are then able to tap into your fat stores for energy. People who eat this way will burn body fat and maintain or increase their muscle mass. This eating plan is what bodybuilders have taught us over the last 30 years. This was long before nutritionists and doctors picked up on it: I learned it from my trainer, and now science has proven that this is the best way to lose fat, gain muscle, and improve health. This technique is hands down the single most important nutritional concept for ultimate leanness and healthy aging.

When your body is presented with too much fuel at any given meal it will store it as body fat for later use. And if you continue to take in too many calories at each meal, your body will never learn how to access this stored fuel, and body fat will continue to accumulate. Constantly feeding your body small meals forces it to process foods *as you eat them* and then use these calories for energy before they can build up as fat in your fat cells. You will also lower your cholesterol levels. In a study reported in the *British Medical Journal* it was shown that people who eat six or more times a day have cholesterol levels that are roughly 5 percent lower than those of less frequent eaters. When you eat larger meals and go for longer periods of time between meals, insulin peaks at higher levels. High peaks of insulin alter fat and cholesterol metabolism—producing higher levels of cholesterol in your blood. Frequent small meals control insulin secretion and prevent these peaks: the result—lower levels of cholesterol. While a 5 percent reduction in cholesterol levels doesn't sound like much, it does have a large impact on your risk for heart disease: It may reduce the chance of coronary artery disease by 10 percent.

The key words to focus on here are: SMALL MEALS. This diet is not a license to eat big meals six times a day, even if you have fully transitioned from bad food choices to good ones. While your health may improve, your waistline certainly won't. You'll see in the next few chapters what small meals look and feel like. I guarantee that it's more than enough food to keep you full all day long.

The whole idea of eating more often to lose weight is one of the toughest concepts for me to get across to my patients: even more than fasting. But the truth is, you can lose weight by eating more often. Once your body gets used to eating every three to four hours you literally become a fat-burning machine. Your body craves nutrients to keep its metabolic processes cranking along at top speed. When I eat one of my small meals my body literally gets hot, and my energy levels increase. The key is to not give your body more calories than it needs at any one time.

However, I know that most men are still eating three big meals, and possibly snacking in between. After the initial fast period, we'll first transition to four meals a day, and after two weeks, you'll move to a five- to six-meal cycle that you'll be able to stay with for the rest of your life.

The Life Plan Diet

I know it's tough for men to follow a diet, which is why I've made the Life Plan Diet almost effortless. There's no calorie counting, and very little measuring. This eating program meets all of the requirements for effectiveness: It is medically sound, flexible, sustainable, and easy to follow for the long term. You'll be able to work this into your day with ease, and if you don't want to share with the world that you're dieting, trust me, no one will notice until they see you are getting healthier and leaner. You can follow the program during work, vacations, business events, and social gatherings.

I have devised four simple nutritional plans that create a stepped dieting approach toward a goal of completely clean eating. These diets promote health and youthful aging because they are low-glycemic and specifically designed to reduce blood pressure and cardiovascular disease while improving overall health and body composition. They focus on whole foods that you can find in any supermarket. Over the course of the next eight weeks, you'll transition from one meal plan to the next. This guarantees success and prevents boredom from eating the same meals over and over again.

When it comes to weight loss there is a vast difference between women and men, not in terms of physiology, but in terms of motivation. I've found that guys are all about learning the program quickly so they end up with bragging rights. You know what I mean: Once you start telling the guys in the office how much you've lost you will gain new respect. So the fastest way I can get you to lose not only pounds, but inches, off your waistline is to focus only on eating. Once you learn how to eat right and avoid the foods that make you fat, you can add to your success by going to the gym. And with this program, every two weeks you'll get to a new, higher level of health that you can tell all your friends about.

You'll begin with the JumpStart program for two weeks. Then, move to the Basic Health Diet for the next two weeks before moving to the final level: the Fat-Burning Diet. The Fat-Burning Diet is more rigorous, but it is absolutely the best way I know to get rid of body fat. You can stay on this diet until you meet your fat-loss goals. Then you can choose to stay on this diet or go back to the Basic Health Diet for maintenance.

If you have already been diagnosed with a heart condition, have a stent, or have a family history of heart disease/stroke, have had bypass surgery, high blood pressure, or other indications that you have vascular disease, stay on the Fat-Burning Diet for two weeks, and then move to the final level: Heart Health. Your goal should be to follow the Heart Health Diet as closely as possible forever. This is a nearly vegan diet that combines low-glycemic eating with a low-fat diet so that you can start reversing blood vessel disease. And if you are having any problems with your sexual health because of documented circulation problems, this is the diet you need to follow forever, as I do.

You will know if the diet is working by three important measurements: the scale, your abdominal girth, and your body fat percentage. By the end of eight weeks you should have dropped several inches from your waist and be well on your way to achieving your ultimate goal.

Follow this eating plan carefully. It is very important that you never skip a meal and that you eat small meals as directed by the portions I've created for you. Make sure that you consume most of your calories before 6:00 p.m. Eating like this sends signals to your body that you are not starving even though you are creating a caloric deficit. You are actually tricking your body and making it a fat-burning machine.

A Real Bonus for Weight Loss: More Sex

- -

Some guys are simply blessed if they have a spouse or partner who will do all their cooking for them. If this is the case you will likely reap many benefits from this diet that go far beyond your weight loss. Studies have proven that couples who diet together see better results. In fact, couples who lose weight together are also more likely to keep the weight off. According to a 2010 Israeli study of spousal dieting, the *wives* of men who were participating in a weight-loss program lost weight themselves—even if they weren't officially dieting.

We also know that women who feel better about their body image enjoy sex more and are interested in having it more frequently. According to a study from 2000 published in the *International Journal of Eating Disorders*, women who are more satisfied with their body reported more sexual activity, increased occurrence of orgasm and initiating sex, and greater comfort undressing in front of their partner, and they enjoy having sex with the lights on and trying new sexual behavior more than those who have a negative body image.

REAL MEN, REAL MOTIVATION: LETTERS FROM MY PATIENTS

Dear Dr. Life,

I want to thank you for helping me achieve the health and conditioning needed to live my vision of an extraordinary life. At age 61 I began my search for a medical program to support my continuing fitness and wellness quest. I had been losing energy and the ability to do the things I love. I didn't want to accept that, move to my couch, telling stories of the past. With your completely integrated program consisting of diet, exercise, supplements, and hormone replacement therapy, my slide to the couch was over. I have followed the program diligently for almost five years and the impact on my quality of life is astounding.

The data from my recent DEXA scan objectively show how I have achieved a physical transformation. With a weight loss of only 1.5 pounds I have lost 33.15 pounds of fat and gained 31.5 pounds of muscle. Dead weight has been replaced with high-energy active weight, and you know me, I've been able to continue the physically demanding activities I enjoy along with trying some new ones. Here are some examples from the last four years:

Diving—Master diver, cold water expert, last January for a month, sailing/diving expedition, 55-foot sailboat with seven others from Argentina to Antarctica across the

Drake Passage. Other major dive trips include the Great Barrier Reef, Coral Sea, Tonga with the Tongan humpback whales, Galapagos twice.

Skiing—As a skier for over 60 years I was thrilled to find myself "zippering" Aspen black diamond moguls last winter. I haven't been able to zipper a mogul run in 20 years.

Hiking—The Inca trails in Peru and an Amazonian jungle trek.

Motorcycling—MotoGP track days (I run midpack with the intermediate riders).

Weight training—I have trained with weights since college as a means of staying in shape. I recently became interested in competition. I found a national-level coach and began training last February. He believes I may be able to rank number one nationally for my age/weight at an upcoming dead lift meet. I'm training Olympic lifts also. This is great fun.

I hesitate using the term "fountain of youth" but for me the shoe fits and I'm wearing it.

Best regards,
AKL

Obstacles You Might Encounter

Occasionally some men reach a plateau in their fat-loss program, and they just can't drop any more body fat. It is rare for my patients not to lose weight on my program, but it's fairly common for them to reach a sticking point just short of their ultimate fat-loss goal. This resistance to fat loss can be caused by several factors, many of which can and should be dealt with before you start your program. That way, you'll ensure success.

Medications. Psychotropic drugs are major impediments to weight loss. These include antidepressants and antianxiety agents. Hormone or hormonelike medications including prednisone are also contributors to limiting weight loss. Cardiovascular, blood pressure, diuretic, and antiarthritic (NSAIDs) drugs can also produce metabolic resistance. If you are taking a medication that you think may be contributing to your inability to lose weight, don't just stop taking it. Talk it over with your doctor and see if an alternative can be used that won't adversely affect your fat-loss efforts.

Your current health. Talk to your doctor to make sure you don't have an underactive thyroid gland, which can cause a lower metabolic rate. Make sure your testosterone levels are healthy. Men with low testosterone have increased abdominal fat. Achieving a healthy testosterone level helps eliminate belly fat.

Extreme stress. If you lead a very stressful life, odds are that it is contributing to your belly fat buildup. If you can't control or reduce the stress in your life by following the suggestions I've made earlier, seek professional help fast. Sometimes, just telling someone that you need help takes a huge burden off your shoulders.

Lack of sleep. Lack of sleep is not commonly thought of as a factor in preventing weight loss, but it is a serious issue. Getting less than seven hours of sleep a night can cause changes in hormones that increase your appetite, which will make following any diet, especially this one, difficult to impossible. In 2012, the *Annals of Internal Medicine* reported on a study that found that lack of sleep alters the biology of fat cells. After just four consecutive nights of less sleep, people's fat cells were less sensitive to insulin, a metabolic change associated with both diabetes and obesity.

You may also eat more the next day, and crave foods high in calories and carbohydrates in order to supply you with the energy you need to get through the day. And as you know, these are exactly the foods that contribute to weight gain. A 2013 study from the University of Colorado recently showed that losing just a few hours of sleep a few nights in a row can lead to almost immediate weight gain. In the course of just one week researchers found that a few late nights affected not only the participants' weight, but their behavior and physiology. The light sleepers ended up eating far more than those who got a full night's sleep, and by the end of the first week the sleep-deprived subjects had gained an average of about two pounds.

CHAPTER 5

Addressing the Elephant in the Room: Men and Drinking

I t would be impossible to write a diet book that addressed men and their belly fat without taking on alcohol consumption head-on. Other diet books may dance around the subject, allowing you to have a drink or two a couple of times a week. Some research even supports the consumption of red wine to lower your risk factors for heart disease. But I'm sorry to say that you just can't have a single alcoholic beverage while you are following the Life Plan Diet. If you want to see your six-pack abs, then you really need to lay off the six-pack of beer, as well as wine, cocktails, and spirits.

If you are a person who can have one drink, or two at the most, then you have pretty good control over your alcohol consumption. But a significant number of men have a problem with alcohol, to some degree or another. And there's a whole spectrum of alcohol abuse that goes from someone who occasionally drinks too much to someone who consistently drinks too much, and people need to be really honest with themselves about where they fall on that spectrum.

But before you throw down the book in sheer disgust, let me just explain to you why, and then maybe you'll come to see things my way:

Alcohol has a unique association with an increased waistline. They don't call it a "beer belly" for nothing. Alcohol is a very concentrated source of calories. That means that it doesn't take much to throw off your caloric intake for the day. An average can of beer has 160 calories, so by the time you've knocked down two you've had as many calories—with no added protein—as a complete meal. Lite beer is not much better: an average 12-ounce "lite" beer has 100 to 130 calories. Cocktails are even worse offenders because they frequently contain lots of sugar in the mixer. Every glass of wine, or shot of spirits, adds up as well.

Alcohol changes the way your liver works. When booze enters your bloodstream, your liver must reduce or stop its metabolism of fats and carbohydrates and many of its other vital functions in order to process it. This causes a buildup of fat in your liver, a decrease in glycogen in your liver and muscles, and an interference with niacin, thiamine, and B vitamin use—all essential for energy production and good health. Simply put: When you drink alcohol, your liver is too busy burning off the alcohol to burn up dietary fat as well, leaving you with a beer belly.

Studies show that alcohol can cause you to feel hungry. There are many reasons why this is true. First, alcohol intake affects hormones that regulate a sense of satiety. Carbohydrate-sensitive people very often crave sweets when they drink. Alcohol is also loaded with carbs, which makes you secrete large amounts of insulin, which makes you hungry.

Alcohol acts as a diuretic, causing you to lose water, which you need in order to get lean, muscular, and healthy. According to researchers at Newcastle University, alcohol acts on the kidneys to make you lose more water than you take in, which is why you need to go to the bathroom so often when you drink. Alcohol also reduces the production of the hormone vasopressin, which tells your kidneys to reabsorb water rather than flush it out through the bladder. With the body's natural signal switched off, the bladder is free to fill up with fluid. This can lead to dehydration, which causes the nausea and headache associated with bad hangovers. It also affects the amount of sugar in your bloodstream, making it that much more difficult for your body to process, which leads to more weight gain and more belly fat.

You're not thinking clearly when you drink. Finally, alcohol affects your brain power so that you have less ability to maintain attention, and that affects your decision-making skills. Ultimately, that can make you less disciplined when it comes to making good food choices, or avoiding food at all.

Now, I'm not saying that I don't enjoy alcohol. In fact, I'm more than willing to tell you that I enjoy it way too much. But I've reached a point in my life where my health is far too important to me to continue making choices that I know negatively affect my body and my brain. So I've learned to lay off booze. It's not been easy, but it's been effective. And as I've said, everything you put in your mouth can either help you or kill you, and that includes alcohol.

The way I avoid alcohol is the same way I avoid trigger foods. Even when I'm out on the town, I focus on my fitness goals and the health of my heart. I remind myself of how I looked and how horrible I felt when I had a big belly. I look at my "before" picture. I think about my wife, my kids, my grandkids, my future, and what their world would be like if I weren't here. And when I put all of this together the last thing I want is to destroy all that I have worked so hard for by having a drink.

This reflective work is beneficial for me, but it may not work for you. If you are having problems with alcohol that you can't handle by yourself, you are definitely not alone. Consider getting professional help from a well-trained addiction specialist. The bottom line is that you need to do whatever it takes to get off alcohol. The payoff is enormous: great health, longevity, leanness, flat belly, better brain, better sexual function, and much more.

Other Drinks to Avoid

Besides alcohol, there are plenty of other beverages that can easily wreck a diet. The truth is, many men consume more calories from what they drink than from what they eat. That may be one of the reasons why you continue to hold on to belly fat even if you think you are eating "clean." Here is a list of all the beverage options you'll be passing on as you follow this program. As with certain foods, you may experience real cravings for many of these, but you'll see that after you've gone without them for a few days, those cravings will subside completely.

Flavored sodas and diet sodas. The average can of soda adds 150 calories to your daily caloric intake, and adds up to 10 teaspoons of sugar to your diet. Many men drink much more than a can a day, especially if they are used to buying those 20-ounce bottles. Carbonated drinks are thought to contribute to obesity as well as diabetes, tooth decay, and weakened bones. They have also been linked to depleting the body of vitamin A, calcium, and magnesium—all nutrients needed for healthy weight loss. Some research suggests that soda's combination of sugar and caffeine can actually make you feel hungrier, signaling the brain to crave extra food.

Diet sodas are not a better option. Sugar substitutes may be low in calories, but they appear to affect the brain the same way as sugar: creating more cravings. According to one study by the University of Texas Health Science Center in San Antonio, diet soda actually enhances weight gain by as much as 41 percent. And diet soda drinkers identified in the famous Framingham Heart Study were at high risk for weight gain and symptoms of the metabolic syndrome.

Fruit/vegetable juice. Compared with soda, 100 percent fruit juice carries more calories and just as much sugar. A glass of juice concentrates all the sugar from several pieces of fruit. When fructose is eaten in a piece of fruit, it enters the body slowly, so the liver has time to convert it into energy. Yet a single glass of apple juice has the fructose of six apples. UC Davis scientist Kimber Stanhope has found that consuming high levels of fructose increases risk factors for heart disease and type 2 diabetes because it is converted into fat by the liver more readily than glucose. Her studies suggest that it doesn't matter whether the fructose is from soda or fruit juice, and that doesn't even take into account fruit juices with added sweeteners, such as cranberry juice or orange drink.

Vegetable juices are a healthier alternative: They are much lower in calories. However, they can be much higher in sodium. My advice is to stick with getting the valuable nutrients found in fruits and vegetables in their whole form, and skip juicing entirely. Even juicing your own fruits and vegetables makes their sugars readily available to the body, and then they are rapidly absorbed from your GI tract into your bloodstream, causing high glucose and insulin levels. This is the exact opposite of what happens when you eat the same ones in their whole form, and the exact opposite of what the Life Plan Diet is all about.

Commercially prepared smoothies and health shakes. Premade smoothies look delicious, and I'm sure they taste great, too. However, you have no control over what goes into them, compared to when you make them in your own home. Prepared smoothies may contain ice cream, honey, or other sweeteners that boost the calorie count.

The Best (and Cheapest) Drink of All: Water

Life Plan Diet Goal: Drink Half
Your Body Weight in Ounces Daily

Along with eating cleanly, you have to drink water to lose belly fat, and I mean lots of it. Water is your most important nutrient. It is involved in every metabolic reaction in your body. Yet most of us don't drink enough. When we are properly hydrated our heart and blood vessels work much better, along with all of our other bodily functions—we think better, our strength and endurance are better, we feel better, we are healthier, and we will live longer. Adequate hydration has the added benefit of helping us eat less by giving us a satisfied feeling—a key ingredient to achieving and maintaining a lean body, especially the gut. Allowing yourself to become even mildly dehydrated can negatively affect your metabolism. In one study from the University of Utah, adults who drank eight or more glasses of water a day burned more calories than those who drank four.

If you want to get really lean and improve your mental and physical performance, I challenge you to drink close to a gallon of water every day. You will be amazed at how much it helps. In one study from Berlin's Franz-Volhard Clinical Research Center, Michael Boschmann, M.D., and his colleagues tracked energy expenditures among men and women who were healthy and not overweight. After drinking approximately 17 ounces of water, the subjects' metabolic rates (the rate at which calories are burned) increased by 30 percent. The increases began within 10 minutes and reached a maximum after 30 to 40 minutes. The study also showed that the increase in metabolic rate differed in men and women. In men, extra water caused them to burn more fat, which fueled their increase in metabolism, whereas in women the additional water increased their breakdown of carbohydrates, which increased their metabolism. The researchers found that up to 40 percent of the increase in calorie burning was caused by the body's attempt to heat the ingested water, suggesting that it's best to drink very cold water. Another 2002 study published in the *American Journal of Epidemiology* found that drinking five or more glasses of water a day reduced the risk of a fatal heart attack by close to 50 percent.

In his book *The Blood Thinner Cure*, Dr. Kenneth R. Kensey writes that most of us go through life in a dehydrated state because we rely on our sensation of thirst as our guide for water consumption. He states that by the time we are thirsty, we are already dehydrated and our blood is too thick, which may be one primary cause of hardening of the arteries, heart attacks, and strokes. I'm not sure I'd go that far, but I do know that a lack of water is the major reason for daytime fatigue. Even mild dehydration will slow your metabolism by as much as 3 percent. A mere 2 percent drop in body water can trigger fuzzy short-term memory, trouble with basic math, and difficulty focusing on the computer screen or on a printed page.

So there you have it, gentlemen: More water translates into more fat burned. If you can increase your water consumption to just 1.5 liters a day (6 cups), you can burn an extra 17,400 calories, for a weight loss of approximately five pounds over the course of a year. So you can burn some serious calories if you drink close to my recommended one gallon (16 cups) a day. You'll be able to accomplish this by drinking small amounts of water throughout the day. For example, drink one tall glass full before you have your first cup of coffee in the morning, then put yourself on a simple schedule of drinking 1½ cups to 3 cups every one to two hours. I find it easier to keep a refillable bottle of water with me throughout the day than to go searching out water sources, not to mention the hundreds of plastic bottles you'll be saving. I have a one-gallon jug of water that I carry around, and I try to consume most of it every day. To mix things up, you can take your water in the form of sparkling water. A few slices of lemon, lime, or even an orange help make cold water easier to drink for me.

The best way to tell that you are getting enough fluids is that you should be making frequent trips to the bathroom, and your urine will be clear, except for when you first go in the morning.

Tea and Coffee: Good for the Brain and the Body

Coffee just may be one of the most important ingredients on the Life Plan Diet. There has been a plethora of research lately that shows how coffee can positively affect both brain and body function. In a 2012 study from the University of South Florida and the University of Miami, blood levels were tested in older adults with mild cognitive impairment, and then re-evaluated two to four years later. Participants with little or no caffeine circulating in their bloodstreams were far more likely to have progressed to Alzheimer's than those whose blood indicated they had been drinking about three cups' worth of caffeine a day. Coffee is also known to be a preventive factor against mild depression.

According to an article in the *New York Times*, other recent studies have linked moderate coffee drinking—15 to 20 ounces a day—with significant health benefits for men. Aside from stimulating your attention and keeping you awake, coffee is connected to a reduction in the risk of developing type 2 diabetes, basal cell carcinoma (the most common skin cancer), prostate cancer, oral cancer, and even Alzheimer's. Other studies directly link coffee consumption to weight loss, and the news has been especially positive for men.

Coffee contains dozens of naturally occurring compounds, including several classes of antioxidants. Caffeine is just one of those naturally occurring substances and is related to increasing energy levels. While some researchers have focused on the caffeine content of coffee as a metabolic booster, others have isolated different nutrients that may play a positive role in weight loss. These compounds are antioxidants known collectively as chlorogenic acids. These acids appear to slow the production of glucose in the body after a meal, by modifying the activity of certain enzymes in the liver. Additionally, the chlorogenic acids cause a more slow and sustained release of glucose into the body after eating, thereby reducing the production of new fat cells. Espresso, made by steam expressing finely ground coffee, is rich in chlorogenic acids, but not in caffeine. Drinking an espresso after eating suppresses glucose production and release, in addition to causing the body to produce more gastric juices, which aids digestion and is thought to enable steady weight loss.

Another study released in 2011 from the New York Obesity Nutrition Research Center, St. Luke's/Roosevelt Hospital Center, identified that consuming mannooligosaccharides (MOS), a complex carbohydrate extracted from coffee, promotes a decrease in body fat. In a double-blind, placebo-controlled weight-loss study it was found that men consuming the MOS beverage had greater loss of body weight, including belly fat, than men consuming the placebo beverage.

For the purposes of your weight loss, or any of the above-mentioned health benefits, it doesn't seem to matter whether you choose caffeinated or decaffeinated coffee. However, some men can't handle too much coffee later in the day because it keeps them up at night. At that point, feel free to switch to decaffeinated. And it goes without saying that any benefit of coffee is going to be more than outweighed if you fill it up with sugar, cream, or high-calorie flavorings. If you can't drink it black, the next-best option is tea.

Tea is also high in nutrients and antioxidants. The darker teas offer the highest antioxidant values. There are three main types of tea, and they are all derived from the same plant, *Camellia sinensis*, yet each has a different taste and appearance. White tea has a higher antioxidant value than green or black tea. It is made from the unfermented young, delicate tea leaves that are covered in fine, white hairs. Black tea is made from the same leaves that have been left on the plant to mature. Green tea is also made from mature leaves, and then fermented.

Green tea is thought to increase metabolism, decrease appetite, improve bone mineral density and strength, and provide more energy for exercise. It is also thought to reduce the absorption of all dietary fats by blocking the production of digestive enzymes that facilitate their absorption. Green tea can help reduce fat by inhibiting the effects of insulin so that sugars are sent directly to the muscles for instant use, instead of being stored as body fat. In one study, participants who regularly consumed hot tea had lower waist circumference and lower BMI than nonconsuming participants. Scientists speculate that regular tea drinking lowers the risk of metabolic syndrome.

Researchers attribute tea's health properties to its antioxidant load. For example, scientists have found that the antioxidants in green tea extract increase the body's ability to burn fat as fuel, which accounts for improved muscle endurance. These same antioxidants might also help protect against cardiovascular and degenerative diseases, including many forms of cancer, may help destroy free radicals, and may protect your skin from the sun's harmful ultraviolet rays.

As we've learned, keeping your body healthy is good for your brain. Tea consumption is thought to be protective against a host of diseases that are known to influence cognitive decline, ranging from heart disease to cancer to allergies and diabetes. It might also be an effective agent in the prevention and treatment of neurological diseases, especially degenerative diseases such as Alzheimer's. Some believe that the polyphenols in green tea may help maintain the parts of the brain that regulate learning and memory. All types of tea contain the nutrient L-theanine, which is thought to stimulate alpha brain waves that are associated with a relaxed but alert mental state, which may increase attention span.

Herbal teas, such as mint or chamomile, are not really tea at all: They are "tisanes" or infusions made from the bark, leaves, and flowers of other plants. While they do not contain theanine or caffeine, they have plenty of other nutrients and health benefits, and are perfectly acceptable options on this diet. They come in myriad flavors, have no calories, and won't keep you up at night. Finally, freshly brewed tea has far more nutrients than anything found in a bottle and is always the preferred option. Many of the popular bottled tea beverages may also be diluted or sweetened, adding unnecessary calories. Worse, their antioxidant levels are 10 to 100 times lower than those in brewed tea.

The bottom line: When you are sick of water, you can switch to a few cups of black coffee or tea each day. Drink it hot or cold. Every cup of coffee or tea counts toward your total water consumption.

The Secret to My Success: Protein Shakes

You'll see in the following meal plans that I'm a big fan of protein shakes. When combined with fruit, they allow me to start the day feeling energized. I also drink them after exercise to help my body recover by restoring muscle glycogen. They also can contribute to muscle repair.

The protein powders used to make shakes come from a variety of sources, such as whey, casein, egg, soy, and milk. These sources may affect your body differently. I've found both whey and casein to be smart choices. I usually drink protein shakes twice a day: a whey protein shake in the morning after my morning workout, and a casein protein shake about 30 minutes before bed.

Whey protein is one of the proteins found in cow's milk. It is isolated from a liquid by-product of cheese production. On the diet you'll mostly be steered toward whey protein shakes, because they contain all of the essential amino acids and have a number of positive health benefits. Whey protein may have anticancer and anti-inflammatory properties, and could possibly act as an effective supplementary treatment for diabetes and heart disease.

In a study published in the *International Journal of Sport Nutrition and Exercise Metabolism*, it was concluded that whey protein provided significantly greater gains in strength and lean body mass and a decrease in fat mass compared to casein. There are three primary types of whey protein: whey protein concentrate (WPC), which contains low levels of fat and high levels of carbohydrates, whey protein isolate (WPI), which has a high percentage of protein by weight, generally over 90 percent, and whey protein hydrolysate (WPH), which is considered a "predigested" form, making it easier for the body to absorb protein. WPH substantially increases insulin, providing more power for your muscles if taken right after you work out.

Casein is a separate type of protein that is also found in milk. Casein is known to have a slow absorption rate, allowing the amino acids in the protein shake to enter the bloodstream slowly. This keeps you feeling full and satisfied for a longer period of time. Casein is an excellent source of protein to consume before bedtime, which is usually the longest interval of time you'll go between meals. This type of shake helps prevent my "nighttime munchies."

There are tons of different protein shakes on the market, including ones that I sell on my website, www.drlife.com (LIFEshakes & LIFEbars). Look for one that has a minimum of 20 grams of protein per scoop.

Either casein or whey protein shakes can be used in the diet. You'll find that they are easy to make and keep you satiated for at least three hours, or until your next meal. They are also perfectly portioned calorie-wise, as well as having the correct protein-fat-carb ratio. This is why I use them almost every day as a meal replacement: They are quick to make, are always fresh, and provide exactly what I need to get through to the next meal. In Chapter 11, I've listed the directions to make my 11 favorite shakes, but you can feel free to create your own once you see the pattern. Remember to avoid adding high-glycemic fruits: Even in small portions these can be dangerous to your success.

In the next chapter, you'll review some of my best tips for staying on track during the diet. With that information and the go-ahead from your doctor, you'll be ready to start the program. Don't wait for the perfect day to start: Today is that day. Just by reading this book you've already taken the important first step to getting your belly fat under control.

CHAPTER 6

The Life Plan Diet Rules of the Road

We are a society of very busy people, and I know that eating right is really hard to do. In order to succeed on this diet, you have to plan. In fact, I find that I have the best results staying on the program when I shop ahead of time so that I have all the food I need on hand for at least a week, and then every morning set up a specific eating plan for the day.

The Life Plan Diet requires very little in the way of specialty foods, but you have to have them on hand at home and where you work. You've got to know exactly what you're going to be eating that day before you go out the door, and you need a contingency plan for those meals that you'll eat at restaurants or other social events. I have found that the best way to make sure I have the right food at home and in my office is to do my grocery shopping online and have it delivered to both locations. That way I'm not tempted to make any "point of purchase" mistakes, like the candy that's sitting right beside the checkout counter. It also guarantees that I have the right foods available to me at my office without my having to remember to bring them with me when I leave home.

The Life Plan Diet Shopping List

It's best to start any diet with a full pantry of the right foods. That will take the guesswork out of what you are going to eat and where you are going to find it. Here is a list of all the foods I used to create the four meal plans and all the recipes. Any of these whole food items (fruits, vegetables, proteins) are acceptable snacks in small increments. For example, you can halve the portions listed to create your own snack.

You'll notice that most of the items on the list are fresh foods. Don't panic: Almost all of them can be eaten raw if you are short on time or don't like to cook. On a typical day I follow the diets exactly as they are written in the meal plans. But as you may find, I can be that limited for only so long. Every couple of weeks when I can't take those meals any longer I start to experiment. I don't go off script: I know I have to stay within the context of the original shopping list. I just swap some of the ingredients on the list below and come up with something new. I also use the recipes in this book as alternative meals, and when I get bored with those, I'll swap out one protein for another, or try a new vegetable.

Sometimes all it takes is spicing up my meals. I can easily add or swap one type of spice for another to create a completely different taste experience. I love spices because they are completely calorie free, and when I use them liberally contain tons of important nutrients. My favorites and the ones I head to first are fresh herbs such as chopped dill, cilantro, and basil. When I can't get to the store to buy fresh, I use the dried varieties or herbs and include some spices as well: Curry seasoning, anise, red pepper flakes, and cinnamon are my go-to choices.

Make a copy of this list and keep it handy so that you have it every time you go grocery shopping. Just by using a shopping list you've given yourself a significant advantage over other dieters: The Hartman Group's Shopping Topography 2012 research showed that fewer than half of primary grocery shoppers (44 percent) normally prepare a shopping list before a trip to the supermarket or grocery store. That means that most shoppers open themselves to all kinds of shopping traps and impulse purchases. If you use this list, and stick to it, you will not buy anything that you don't need to eat.

I've also included the nutritional information for each item on the shopping list so that you can make good choices when you are swapping out one item for another, and compare within each category what the best options are for you.

For each of the meals throughout the book, you'll see that I have given you the amount (weight or volume) of each food item. But I must tell you, I never weigh my food. I simply eyeball each portion and follow these simple guidelines. When you are eating healthy foods you will lose more weight only by eating less, especially at the beginning of a program. I always make sure I err on the side of making each serving a little smaller than I think it should be.

- A four-ounce portion of animal protein is roughly the size of your palm (width, length, and thickness) . . . be sure you don't include your fingers and thumb.

- The right amount of vegetables is roughly what you can hold in your cupped hand. However, you have a lot of leeway with veggies. You can always eat more veggies without adding too many calories, as long as you eat them without adding extra fats. Vegetables add lots of nutrients and fiber and do a great job keeping you feeling full until your next meal.

- A carbohydrate portion, like a yam or wild rice, is slightly smaller than a clenched fist. If you have a lot of belly fat to lose, estimate using a smaller fist as a guide.

- For packaged foods that are measured by volume, just measure it out in comparison to its package. The next time you'll know about how much you need for a serving without going to all of the trouble of measuring it again.

Food	Typical Serving Size	Calories	Protein Grams	Fat Grams	Carb Grams
PROTEINS					
Almonds	22 nuts	153	6	13	5
Adzuki beans	1 cup	295	17	0	57
Beans, white	1 cup	299	19	1	56
Beef, lean	4 oz	193	30	3	0
Black beans, canned	2 oz	60	4	0	11
Black bean veggie burger (Morningstar brand)	1 patty	120	11	4	13
Casein protein powder	1 scoop	120	24	10	4
Cashews	28 nuts	157	9	12	5
Cheese, shredded	1 oz	81	1	6	1
Cheese, soy	1 oz	70	2	5	2
Chicken breast, boneless/skinless	4 oz	164	25	6	0
Chicken broth, reduced sodium	1 cup	17	2	0	1
Cottage cheese, low-fat	1 cup	81	14	1	3
Cream cheese, low-fat	1 tbs	23	1	2	1
Egg whites	5 egg whites	86	18	0	2
Flounder	4 oz	132	27	1	0
Garbanzo beans (chick peas)	1 cup	269	15	4	45
Greek yogurt, low-fat	1 cup	130	23	0	9
Halibut	4 oz	178	34	4	0
Hemp seeds	1 oz	162	10	13	2
Hummus	1 tbs	50	1	3	5
Kidney beans	1 cup	225	15	0	40
Mackerel	4 oz	230	21	4	0
Mahi mahi	4 oz	157	33	1	0
Milk, 1%	1 cup	102	8	2	13
Milk, skim	1 cup	86	8	0	12
Orange roughy	4 oz	100	21	0	0
Peanut butter, natural reduced-fat	2 tbs	200	9	12	1
Pine nuts	1 cup	909	18	92	18
Pork loin, lean/boneless	1 chop	286	40	13	0
Salmon	4 oz	240	27	15	0

Food	Typical Serving Size	Calories	Protein Grams	Fat Grams	Carb Grams
Sardines	1 small	25	3	1	0
Scallops	5 small	26	5	0	1
Shrimp	4 oz	55	11	0	0
Smoked salmon	4 oz	133	21	5	0
Soy yogurt, unsweetened	1 cup	130	10	6	7
Steak, T-bone, visible fat removed	4 oz	200	29	8	0
String cheese, low-fat	2 pieces	120	14	5	1
Tilapia	4 oz	148	31	3	0
Tofu, low-fat, extra-firm	4 oz	120	16	3	8
Trout	4 oz	170	24	7	0
Tuna, fresh or frozen	4 oz	147	34	1	0
Tuna, canned in water	4 oz	122	26	1	0
Turkey breast, boneless/skinless	4 oz	153	34	1	0
Turkey jerky	1 oz	100	19	1	1
Turkey luncheon meat, nitrate/nitrite free	4 oz	120	26	2	2
Vegan sausage links, low-sodium	1 link	70	11	0	0
Walnuts	14 halves	185	4	18	4
Whey protein	1 scoop	110	22	1	1

GRAINS

Food	Typical Serving Size	Calories	Protein Grams	Fat Grams	Carb Grams
Basmati rice, brown uncooked	1 cup	160	4	0	35
Brown rice uncooked	¾ cup	216	5	2	45
Bulgur wheat dry uncooked	1 cup	479	17	2	106
Cabbage, red	1 cup	13	0	0	3
Ezekiel 4:9 sprouted grain bread	1 slice	80	4	1	15
Granola, low-fat	½ cup	186	4	3	39
Oatmeal, steel-cut	¼ cup dry	170	7	3	29
Oats, rolled	½ cup	303	13	5	52
Quinoa	½ cup	114	4	0	21
Rice flour	5.5 oz	578	9	2	127
Seitan wheat protein	3 oz.	150	18	1	3
Tempeh	1 cup	320	31	18	16
Wild rice, cooked	1 cup	166	6	1	35

Food	Typical Serving Size	Calories	Protein Grams	Fat Grams	Carb Grams
FRUITS					
Apples	1 large	116	1	0	30
Blueberries	½ cup	41	1	0	11
Cherries	1 cup	194	2	1	49
Grapefruit	½ grapefruit	52	1	0	13
Grapes, black	40	64	1	0	16
Lemon	½ fruit	8	0	0	3
Nectarines	1	59	1	0	14
Olives	¼ cup	82	1	9	2
Oranges	1 medium	62	1	0	16
Peaches	1 medium	59	1	0	14
Pears	1 large	121	1	1	32
Raspberries	1 cup	65	1	0	5
Strawberries	1 cup	46	1	1	11
Tangerines	1	40	1	0	10
VEGETABLES					
Artichokes	2 hearts	45	3	0	10
Asparagus	8 spears	26	1	0	3
Avocados	(⅓ medium)	91	5	8	1
Black-eyed peas	1 cup	130	4	0	27
Bok Choy	1 cup	20	3	0	3
Broccoli	1 cup	55	4	0	11
Brussels sprouts	1 cup	38	3	0	8
Carrots	1 cup	80	0	0	19
Cauliflower	1 cup	25	2	0	5
Celery	2 stalks	5	2	0	0
Cucumbers	1 cup	14	0	0	6
Edamame, shelled	1 cup	250	20	6	18
Eggplant	1 cup	35	0	0	9
Green beans	1 cup	44	2	0	10
Iceberg lettuce	2 cups	32	6	1	2
Kale	2 cups	67	4	1	13

Food	Typical Serving Size	Calories	Protein Grams	Fat Grams	Carb Grams
Mushrooms	1 cup	16	4	0	4
Onions, white	½ small	15	0	0	4
Red bell peppers	1 cup	38	2	0	8
Snap peas	1 cup	41	3	0	7
Spinach	2 cups	16	0	2	1
Squash	1 cup	82	2	0	22
String beans	1 cup	44	2	0.1	10
Swiss chard	1 leaf	7	1	0	1
Sweet potatoes, yam	Fist size	157	2	0	40
Tomatoes	1 cup diced	32	2	0	8
Yams	Fist size	164	3	0	40
Zucchini	1 cup diced	80	6	0	0

CONDIMENTS

Food	Typical Serving Size	Calories	Protein Grams	Fat Grams	Carb Grams
Capers	1 tbs	2	0	0	0
Cilantro	¼ cup	1	0	0	0
Distilled white vinegar	0.5 oz	2	0	0	0
Garlic	1 tbs	13	0	0	3
Jalepeno pepper	3 oz	27	1	1	6
Low-fat vinaigrette salad dressing	1 tbs	43	0	4	2
Mustard	1 tbs	0	0	0	0
Olive oil mayonnaise	1 tbs	45	0	4	2
Ranch dressing, low-fat	1 tbs	45	0	4	4
Relish, sweet	1 tbs	20	0	0	5
Salsa	½ cup	70	4	0	15
Soy sauce, low-sodium	2 tsp	6	0	0	1
Vegetable broth	1 cup	15	0	0	3

FATS

Food	Typical Serving Size	Calories	Protein Grams	Fat Grams	Carb Grams
Canola oil	1 tbs	124	0	14	0
Nonfat cooking spray	1 spray	0	0	0	0
Olive oil, extra-virgin	1 tsp	43	0	5	0
Sesame seed oil	1 tbs	120	0	14	0

If there is anything on this list that you are allergic to or simply don't like and won't eat, by all means choose something else. I've chosen these foods because they are all high in nutrients with the lowest amount of calories, and quite frankly, I like them. From the above list, the following are some of my favorite foods and why they were important to include (so if you can, make an extra effort to at least try them, unless you have a known food allergy):

Blueberries: A super food if there ever was one. These antioxidant-rich berries prevent inflammation, promote better thinking, and are one of the most powerful antioxidants.

Broccoli: This nutrient-rich veggie helps stimulate the immune system and protect against damage. It contains vitamins A and C, a healthy amount of fiber, and glutathione and sulforaphane (anticancer agents).

Cabbage: Contains glutathione, which prevents cellular damage caused by free radicals.

Eggs: Eggs are a perfect protein and an excellent choice. Eggs have gotten a bad rap because they have fairly high levels of saturated fat and cholesterol, which are thought to contribute to heart disease. According to Thomas Behrenbeck, M.D., Ph.D., a cardiologist with the Mayo Clinic, while chicken eggs are high in cholesterol, eating four egg yolks or fewer on a weekly basis hasn't been found to increase your risk of heart disease. And because eggs can be eaten without any additional fat (think hard- or soft-boiled) and the rest of my diet is very low in foods that increase cholesterol, they are still on my must-have list. If you already have been diagnosed with heart disease and you are still leery, use only the egg whites, which contain all the protein and none of the cholesterol.

Ezekiel bread: This is one of the very few processed foods that I'll allow. This bread doubles as a complete protein that closely parallels the protein found in milk and eggs. In fact, the protein quality is so high, it is 84.3 percent as efficient as the highest recognized source of protein—and it's made from all-vegetable sources. It is also rich in vitamins, minerals, and natural fiber, without added fat. Best of all, it actually tastes good. However, don't look for it in the bread aisle: It's often kept in the refrigerated cases of health food stores and most supermarkets.

Grapefruit: Packed with vitamin C and flavonoids to support your immune system and reduce insulin levels. They also have many fewer calories than oranges or orange juice. A 2006 study conducted at the Nutrition and Metabolic Research Center at Scripps Clinic found that eating half a grapefruit before each meal helped people drop more than three pounds over 12 weeks.

Grapes: A great snack when eaten frozen. They keep my fingers and mind busy so that

I don't think about eating other sweets that are worse for me. And I can't eat very many or eat them very fast when they are frozen.

Mushrooms: Excellent choice to boost your immune response. Mushrooms of all varieties are rich in the mineral selenium as well as B vitamins (riboflavin and niacin).

Nuts: People who snack on nuts tend to be slimmer than those who don't. A study from Purdue University found that when a group of 15 normal-weight people added about 500 calories worth of peanuts to their regular diet, they consumed less at subsequent meals. Walnuts contain omega-3 fatty acids; pecans can reduce heart disease risks; and almonds are high in healthy fats along with vitamin E, vitamin B, niacin, and riboflavin.

Olive oil or light mayonnaise: Great-tasting, with more than half the calories of other brands. Very little saturated fat (0.5 gram) and no trans fats or sugar. It takes very little to add great flavor to boiled egg whites, vegetables, and some meats.

Peanut butter: One of my very favorite snacks because it's an excellent protein source. Read labels very carefully and choose one that has absolutely nothing added besides roasted peanuts. Along with yogurt it's one of the few foods that will keep you feeling satisfied and help you burn calories.

Pears: The fruit that contains the most fiber of any fruit, which means that they aid digestion, decrease blood sugar levels, and also fill you up. Apples are another good, low-glycemic choice that come in second in terms of fiber.

Poultry (turkey and chicken): Power foods that are high in protein and have very little fat.

Protein bars: Some men eat protein bars like they are cookies. The typical man may eat two or three of these bars and end up taking in way too many calories. These bars may be high in protein, but they are typically also high in sugar. In my personal experience, the bars don't satisfy you in terms of being a full meal replacement, but many have the same number of calories as a complete meal on the Life Plan Diet. Worst of all, they cause a lot of bloating. Some manufacturers recommend eating the bars with a full glass of water because of the fiber content.

Protein bars are great if you're traveling and you need something to eat that will keep you out of a restaurant. Just make sure that you're choosing one that is both low in sugar and high in protein, and doesn't have a long list of harmful ingredients. In addition to my LIFEbars, the following are the companies I prefer: Quest Nutrition, BioTrust, Perma Lean Protein bar, Rise Bar, Simply Whey bar, and YouBar, which allows you to build your own bars right on their website (www.youbars.com). This feature is perfect for men with food allergies: You can custom order exactly what you like for as little as six bars at a time, based on specific ingredients as well as specific nutrients, including an accurate count of protein grams.

Red bell peppers: Loaded with vitamin C (more than twice as much as other vitamin C–rich veggies/fruits) and beta carotenes, which give the red-orange pigment, red and orange peppers protect cells from free radical damage and enhance immune system function.

Spinach: Spinach helps new cell production and DNA repair and strengthens your body's immune system because it is high in the B vitamin folate as well as vitamin C and fiber.

Sweet potatoes/yams: Another beta carotene–rich food, sweet potatoes are high in fiber and are a great source of vitamin A. Substitute a yam every time you have a hankering for a potato.

Whey protein: I use this for my shakes, and sometimes in my oatmeal.

Yogurt: Yogurt's live/active cultures help you battle colds by activating your immune system. According to a 2011 study from the Harvard School of Public Health, yogurt is at the top of a very short list of foods that actually increase metabolism. Try higher-protein Greek yogurt since it's creamier and triple-strained to remove the whey.

Choosing the Best Fruits and Vegetables

Most vegetables are considered low-glycemic, so if your favorite isn't on this list, feel free to swap it whenever you want. The only exception is corn and white potatoes. Those are high-glycemic and are not included on this diet. In the same Harvard study citing the benefits of nuts and protein, potatoes came down as the single worst food culprit. The study showed that every additional serving of potatoes people added to their regular diet each day made them gain roughly one-quarter pound of body fat every year. French fries and potato chips were just as bad for you as mashed, baked, or boiled potatoes.

The following list includes the fruits that are considered low-glycemic. As a general rule, you'll be avoiding high-glycemic fruits. These include tropical fruits, which are exactly what you imagine: fruits that grow in hot climates mostly outside of the mainland United States. This list includes pineapple, banana, pomegranates, guava, mango, papaya, and fresh figs. Dried fruits are also a bad choice because they are extremely high in sugar, and you may end up eating large quantities of them because they don't bulk up when their water content is removed. Dehydrated or freeze-dried alternatives would be a much better choice.

The best fruit choices can be enjoyed every day:

- Apples

- Apricots

- Berries (any type)

- Grapefruit

- Grapes

- Melons

- Nectarines

- Oranges

- Peaches

- Pears

- Plums

My War Against the Food Manufacturers

In my opinion, the food manufacturers are in large part responsible for the obesity epidemic in America today. In 1985 the National Heart, Lung, and Blood Institute through its Cholesterol Education Program advised us that to maintain a heart-healthy diet we needed to cut our intake of fat and cholesterol and replace it with carbohydrate calories, mostly from whole grains. The food manufacturers jumped on this and started the massive proliferation of the countless wheat products we have today. This marked the beginning of our ever-expanding waistline along with heart disease and type 2 diabetes.

Wheat now dominates our daily diet in a way that it never did when I was growing up. If you want to get rid of belly fat then you must avoid all processed wheat products and other packaged goods produced by food manufactures. You'll see in Part Two that on my diet virtually no packaged foods are allowed. You'll be shopping the perimeter of the grocery store where the fresh foods are located, so you won't be tempted to buy anything that you can't eat. However, even our best plans go awry. There are surprise trips, late nights in the office, and so on. You may find yourself stuck somewhere without your best food options, and you have to eat something.

Once you learn how to read nutritional labels you can begin to make better food choices on the fly. You'll also begin to realize what is in the foods that you have been eating, and how food manufacturers claim that certain foods are "healthy" dependent on their serving sizes. In addition to the nutrition label, products may display certain information or health claims on packaging. These claims are not necessarily regulated and do not have to adhere to industry standards—another reason I just stick to buying foods in their rawest, most unprocessed, and freshest forms.

The Food and Drug Administration mandated that food manufacturers add nutrition labels to all packaged foods, including supermarket meats, in 1994. The nutrition facts label currently appears on more than 6.5 billion food packages. The most useful information is the breakdown of saturated fats, trans fats, sodium, calories, and serving size. Avoid foods that are high in sugar, low in fiber, high in fructose corn syrup, and high in saturated fat. My rule is that if a processed food has more than one gram of sugar or any high-fructose corn syrup, I just don't buy it. I will only purchase foods that have 0 to 0.5 grams of saturated fat, and no trans fats. The more fiber it has, the better. And remember, the more processed a food is the more it will promote belly fat and poor health.

Making It Work

There are very few people I know who are naturally lean and can eat whatever they want. My patients who are lean work at it all the time. And they all tell me the same thing: "I plan ahead."

The late Coach John Wooden's adage "If you fail to plan you plan to fail" holds very true in basketball as well as in creating a successful fat-loss program. This might mean preparing meals in advance and taking them with you so that you don't find yourself hungry and trapped, pulling into a fast-food restaurant and eating a high-calorie, high-fat, low-nutrition meal.

Here are some of my best planning tips and key rules I try to follow daily that really help me stay on track. They can play an essential role in helping you achieve your goals of leanness, increased energy, and great health. What's more, they'll help make the Life Plan Diet easy to follow:

1. Cook enough protein and veggies to have meals ready in the fridge for several days.

2. Always pack lunches and snacks to take with you, whether you are going on a short vacation or on a business trip for a couple of days.

3. Have meal replacement bars and/or shakes on hand.

4. Plan your meals according to your day's activities—heavier meals before a workout, smaller meals before a nap or watching TV.

5. Always carry water with you—a no-calorie way to fill yourself up before, after, and between meals.

6. Make a list of the reasons you want to lose body fat and keep it off forever. Laminate it, carry it in your wallet, and refer to it frequently.

7. Take a "before" picture of yourself with your cell phone and look at it once a day. You'll be surprised just how quickly your body will begin to change.

8. Photocopy your shopping list and keep a copy in your wallet, or type it into your cell phone as a permanent reminder of what you need to buy.

9. Don't eat unless you are sitting at a table. Your car doesn't count as a table.

10. Avoid eating fast. Savor every bite. Try to spend at least 15 minutes eating each and every meal. You can make yourself slow down by taking 20 chews per bite and putting less food on your fork for every mouthful.

11. Use a small plate. It makes you feel and think that you're eating more food than you really are.

12. Don't consume any calories for at least two hours before you go to bed.

13. Make getting a good night's sleep a priority.

14. Avoid buffets and other places where there are many food choices—the more food choices you have the more you will eat too much of the wrong foods.

15. No finger foods—ever.

16. Keep bad food out of your house.

17. Look away from the television when food commercials are thrown at you.

18. Don't eat bread when you're on the road or any time you're away from home.

19. Stay out of the kitchen between meals.

20. Don't miss any meals. Eat every two to three hours.

Tips for Fasting

The short fast that begins the program taught me what it actually felt like to be hungry, and I realized that it was a feeling that I could handle. Yet as strong as my willpower was, I had to attend a family barbecue on my first fast day. I'd be lying if I didn't admit that I just could not stop thinking about the hamburgers and chicken I saw and smelled on the grill. I knew I had to remove myself from the situation, so I just got up, grabbed a bottle of water, and told my wife that I had to take a walk. Once I got away from the party, I was able to get the idea of food out of my head.

But the real lesson was what I learned about myself. Normally I would've eaten about 1,000 to 1,500 calories at that meal, throwing out the diet entirely, and really gotten into the event. There's no doubt I would've had at least two hamburgers and my favorite side dishes: macaroni salad and potato salad. If I was feeling motivated about staying on my diet, I might have chosen to "be social," throwing away the buns and choosing one salad instead of two, and still have eaten 500 calories. But this time I didn't eat anything. It was an eye-opener for me that I could really do this, and it wasn't nearly as hard as I thought it would be. It felt great that I was able to win this battle.

There were other times on the fast when I had to distract myself—by stretching, doing some kind of exercise, walking, closing my eyes for a five-minute power nap, going to my tablet or phone and playing games—from thinking about food. I also had to keep drinking water to ensure that I wouldn't dehydrate and get a headache. But I realized that these are perfectly acceptable techniques to use when fasting or even when you get a craving: Just take a break and focus on something else. Or drink a large glass of water or a cup of hot coffee. In a few minutes, the craving will go away and again, you'll win the battle.

Avoid Obstacles When Eating Out

The trend today is healthy eating: organic, locally grown, artisanal, and sustainable foods. Restaurants have learned to cater to your needs instead of forcing you to eat what they prepare. What's more, even fast-food joints are offering a variety of healthier choices on the menu, such as salads, grilled chicken dishes, smoothies, and fresh fruit options.

When Annie and I first met, we used to go out for lunch or dinner all the time, each ordering our own appetizers, main course, and dessert. When I started my transformation, we switched our habits: We'd share an appetizer and then each order an entrée, and then share dessert. That worked, but I realized the portions served at restaurants are typically too large: I'd end up eating way too many calories as I enjoyed my meal. Now we each order an appetizer and share one entrée. We find that this provides plenty of food to satisfy our hunger, and at the same time we don't leave the table feeling overfull. On the rare occasions that we do eat dessert, we'll share one, with the goal to leave half of it on the plate. I've got to tell you, however, this rarely works, so the best plan is no dessert.

The next time you're dining out remember the following and you'll be able to stick very close to the Life Plan Diet:

- ALWAYS politely pass on the bread basket.

- ALWAYS ask for water, and drink at least a whole glass before you eat anything. This will help curb your appetite and aid in digesting whatever follows.

- SKIP carbonated beverages regardless of whether they are sweetened with sugar or sugar substitute. Tea or coffee, hot or iced, are acceptable options, as long as you can drink them unsweetened. Carbonated, unflavored water (mineral water, seltzer, club soda) is acceptable, however.

- PASS on ordering any alcohol. Beer, wine, and hard spirits will derail your success, especially at the beginning of the diet.

- ALWAYS order a fish entrée, and ask for the sauce to be served on the side or not at all—even if the restaurant doesn't list a sauce on the menu. Grilled chicken is your next-best option. If the waitperson says (and I've had this happen), "We can't do substitutions," then very matter-of-factly explain that this is not a substitution at all, just a healthier choice, and you don't want the sauce or butter added. If it's still an issue, just ask to speak with the manager. It's amazing how much attention that grabs.

- ALWAYS order salad dressings served "on the side" and use sparingly.

- BEWARE of salad entrées: They often contain as many calories as a more traditional entrée. Skip salads that contain cheese, bacon, fried chicken or fish, and creamy dressings.

- CONSIDER vegetarian entrées carefully: They can be just as fattening as animal proteins. Avoid high-calorie options that are smothered in cheese or creamy sauces.

- NEVER order any type of sandwich-style entrée. Many times I order a sandwich "without the bread" if there is nothing else on the menu that I can eat.

- NEVER order cream-based soups, breaded or fried foods, or even fried vegetables.

- NEVER order pasta-based entrées: The carb-to-protein ratio will never match what I recommend.

- ALWAYS ask to substitute a side salad with a vinaigrette dressing, or steamed vegetables in place of French fries, potatoes, or white rice UNLESS sweet potatoes or brown rice are available.

- IF YOU CAN'T SHARE, TAKE HOME HALF: If the portion looks larger than what you've been eating at home following this program, ask the waiter to bring you a "to go" box and take half off your plate before you start eating.

- NEVER choose buffets or fast-food restaurants where there are too many options and most of them are bad—the more food choices you have the more likely it is that you will eat too much of the wrong foods.

- NEVER start a meal with finger foods—nachos, fried cheese sticks, potato skins, even peel-and-eat shrimp. If you can't use a knife and fork, you are more likely to overindulge.

- SKIP dessert, unless they are serving fresh berries. Sorry, no cream.

The Life Plan Diet Goes to a Party

Social events and holidays will inevitably come up and will test your willpower. To control your eating when you are at parties, you must create a strategy before you get there and then stick to it. Rehearse in your mind just how you are going to deal with the foods and beverages offered.

First, never leave your home feeling hungry. Fifteen minutes before I leave for any event I have a rounded tablespoon of Metamucil in an eight-ounce glass of water. Metamucil is psyllium, a nonsoluble fiber that mixes with the foods you are about to eat, thereby slowing the speed of digestion and the release of sugars into your bloodstream. This really slows the entire process of eating way down and can give you the extra edge you need for staying in control when you are confronted with some of your favorite foods—and drinks.

If your host insists on having you try something that has been specially prepared for the party, just let him or her know that a doctor has you on a special nutrition plan to correct a potentially lethal medical condition (fatness—but you don't have to say that). Then, eat only the healthiest options and avoid your trigger foods. Stay away from the passed hors d'oeuvres: You can't keep track of how many you've eaten, because they do not fill a plate. If you start obsessing over one of your trigger foods, tell someone about the diet: This will make it less likely that you will allow yourself to get caught shoving something you shouldn't into your mouth.

Appoint yourself as the designated driver so that you won't be tempted to drink. And, if all else fails and you are having a miserable time, graciously thank your host and leave early.

REAL MEN, REAL MOTIVATION: TROY AND DAVE

Troy Oswalt and Dave Moody are patients of mine who have appeared with me on the *Dr. Phil* show; first in July 2012 and then again in August 2013. They have both made incredible journeys into good health and great physical shape, and I couldn't be more proud to share their stories with you.

I first met Troy when he was 42: He had just suffered a heart attack. This kind of guy is my favorite type of patient, because I know that if I can get him to follow my program, I can totally reverse his health. At six foot one and 260 pounds, Troy was lucky to be alive, but he was very lethargic, unmotivated, and tired all the time. Worst of all, high-calorie food was an inescapable part of his life. He is a chef at one of the large casinos in Las Vegas, working in the banquet department, surrounded by food. On top of all the meals he had access to during an 8- to 10-hour shift, he'd be too tired to start cooking for his family and would bring home fast food for dinner.

Troy knew that he had to kick his bad eating habits and start exercising if he wanted to live to see his kids graduate, even from elementary school. And in one year he did just that. He's already down 70 pounds and making the right decisions about food, not only for himself, but for the entire family. He's also using my Life Plan Diets at work, cooking healthier meals for the employee dining room. His peers were motivated by his great results, and now they're eating healthier as well and dropping fat.

But don't wait for the medical wake-up call to start improving your health. I see lots of guys who've just simply had enough. For example, Dave was 53 years old and 245 pounds and was sick and tired of being tired all the time. He first came to see me at the tail end of the Great Recession: He is a banker, and on a scale between 1 and 10, he told me that his stress level on a typical workday was about a 7. He also told me that whenever he was really stressed he'd head straight for comfort foods and sleep, just trying to get through the day. Exercise was not a part of his life at all, and he was completely out of shape.

Just one year later, he tells me—and anyone else who'll listen—that he's feeling fantastic. His medical tests show that his body is working as if he were 20 years younger: He's lost 50 pounds and has regained his energy. As the economy picks up things are starting to get easier at work, and his improved energy allows him to get more accomplished each day. Combining this with daily exercise and the right diet, even Dave is surprised to see that his stress has diminished.

Dave's motivation comes from keeping an eye on his "before" pictures that he carries in his wallet. That's the same strategy I used when I first got into shape, and I still use it to this day. When I look at those pictures I can hardly believe that was me. There's no way I'm going back to be that old 57-year-old man, when I can be 75 and look and feel as good as I do.

So what are you waiting for? Snap a shot of yourself and get with the Life Plan Diet. You'll be amazed at the results, and just like Troy and Dave, you'll be motivated to keep going until you find your best self.

The Life Plan Diet Is Forever

I know that you are going to find the diet challenging, and I hope that you can embrace the challenge. The changes that you are going to experience are going to be nothing short of monumental. Within a few weeks you are going to feel better physically and mentally. You'll have more energy to do the things you enjoy. Your anxiety may lessen and your mood will improve. You might find that you are sleeping better at night, and wake up feeling rested and refreshed in the morning. And you won't be the only one to notice these changes: Prepare yourself for lots of positive feedback from your coworkers, friends, and family. They'll notice your transformation, and their positive energy will keep you motivated.

So let's start talking about the long haul. I can't say this any more clearly: The Life Plan Diet is forever. I've outlined the next eight weeks in Part Two, but you will see the results that I've been able to achieve only when you stay the course forever. That means every day of every week. If you can do this, you'll accomplish more than most men ever do. And that's going to be something for you to brag about.

Many popular diets allow you to take a day off from eating right, but I've found that this so-called free day isn't free at all. Unfortunately, it doesn't take much to go back to poor eating habits, and what may start as an occasional "treat" may quickly turn into a disappointing return of belly fat. If you are reading this book because you have always had a problem with control (like most of us) and if you recognize that you're especially vulnerable to trigger foods, then you simply can't afford a free day.

In all honesty, I cheat every once in a while. But I know that if I take a free day I'll lose control for a whole lot longer. Instead, when I mess up and eat something that I shouldn't, I don't beat myself up. I just move along, and the very next meal I'll get right back on track. So instead of thinking about a free day, I have a "free" meal once a week, at the most. I try very hard to make sure that I completely avoid my trigger foods that cause me to lose control, even during those free meals.

Now that you have a full understanding of how this diet works and what you need to have before you begin, let's get started on the fast. If you make a mistake and step off the path, don't wait for "the end of the week" or the start of business on Monday to get back on the program: You don't have this luxury. The more time you spend off track, the harder it will be to get back on.

Once you have reached your goals, continue to monitor your body fat percentage, muscle mass, and strength, and see your doctor so that he or she can track all of your biomarkers for disease. Get new bathing suit photos of yourself every month and post them right next to your "before" photo on your refrigerator door, or in your wallet. Cycle through the JumpStart program every eight weeks to revisit the fast and reset your internal systems if you found that it was motivating. You can also visit my website (www.drlife.com) for tons of interviews with experts and my weekly podcasts about fitness, healthy aging, tricks about staying on track, short PowerPoint talks, and much more.

PART TWO

THE LIFE PLAN DIET

CHAPTER 7

The JumpStart Diet

Weeks 1 and 2

The Life Plan JumpStart Diet begins with a 36-hour fast in which you don't consume any calories. You just drink plenty of water, black coffee, or tea (no sugar, no milk/cream). I have learned that a 36-hour fast is ideal, because in that time I am able to gain a better understanding of how my eating affects my physical health and my mood. I suggest that you have your last meal on Friday night and then begin eating again on Sunday morning as I describe below.

I also believe from my own experience that occasional fasting after eating your last meal for the day at three o'clock and not eating until the next morning is also beneficial, especially if you've reached a plateau and you just can't get your weight to come down any more. The fasting will increase your ability to burn fat and help you bust through that plateau.

My Experience Fasting

I fasted for the first time in the summer of 2013. I had never fasted before in my life. For the past 15 years I've been a staunch believer in the importance of eating every two to three hours, so this was a whole new experience for me. Frankly, I didn't know if I could do it.

I made the commitment to the fast because I'd been hearing a lot about fasting, its benefits, and how it might fit into a responsible fat-loss program. I started my fast following a weeklong family reunion with my kids and grandkids. I had gotten myself way off course. I did not drink any alcohol, but I ate badly. Even though I continued to exercise, I knew I had gained a lot of weight while I was there, which was another reason why fasting seemed so appealing to me. I decided to try a two-day fast so I could make sure that my body was fully engaged in ketosis.

I ate my last meal on Sunday night. Monday morning I woke up and went to the gym to work out. I continued throughout the day drinking plenty of water and not eating anything. I would have intermittent hunger pangs, and I just ignored them. Instead, I would just find something else to distract me, such as doing my abdominal stretches. In the past I've found that stretching is a great way for me to get rid of cravings, and it worked just as well with my hunger pangs.

I was able to get through the first day without a whole lot of trouble. I actually felt energized, and I definitely didn't feel tired or sluggish. That evening I kept myself busy in the house so that I was too distracted to think about food. I assumed that I would have a lot of trouble sleeping that first night, but I didn't. Actually, I had no trouble sleeping at all.

Tuesday morning I skipped the gym and went to a doctor's appointment with my wife. While I was waiting I continued to drink coffee. When we came home that afternoon I continued to just drink water and coffee and some tea. I experienced a little bit of a headache off and on throughout the day, but nothing I couldn't handle. I still felt energetic. I carried on with my normal activities, for the most part. I did have more hunger pangs Tuesday afternoon than I did on the first day and a half.

That evening we went to a family barbecue, which I talked a bit about earlier in this book. Hamburgers and hot dogs were cooking on the grill, as well as many of my favorite foods—potato salad, macaroni and cheese, macaroni salad—that are usually very hard for me to resist. I got to the point where I just couldn't stop thinking about these foods. I could smell the food and see how good it looked on the grill, and after just a couple of minutes, I told Annie that I had to go for a walk. I grabbed a bottle of water and left. By the time I came back, they'd finished cooking, and even the dishes were done and the food was put away. Without the ability to look at food or other people eating, I was good the rest of that night.

Wednesday morning the fast officially ended. I got out of bed and had three eggs and a chicken breast for breakfast. I thought that I would be starving and anxious to eat a lot of food, but in reality it was really hard for me to eat that much. After breakfast I went back to bed and slept for another three hours. The second time around I got up, ate some more, and then the rest of the day was fine. When I weighed myself, I had lost 11.5 pounds, most of which was water. The fast also had a profound psychological impact, and I was reinvigorated to continue my fat-loss program.

When I woke up Thursday morning, I was back to my normal routine with exercise, and I've been feeling fine ever since. Here I am, 75 years old and had never fasted in my life, and I accomplished my goal. Once I resumed eating, my energy levels came back, and I'm just as strong and my endurance is just as good.

Before the fast I really thought that there were some men who just couldn't do this challenge, and that I would be one of them. Typically, I go around feeling a little bit hungry all the time: That's my way of keeping track of my metabolism, because if I'm hungry I know that my body is burning fat for fuel. I also know that I have a consumption disorder. So going without food for two whole days was a massive, major achievement for me.

I also found that fasting actually reset my hunger thermostat. During the fast, and for the few days after it, I wasn't near as hungry as I typically am. Most of the time I didn't think about food and I didn't even think about hunger, and by the end I really felt energized.

How to Fast and Return to Food Safely
- -

Your last meal before the fast begins will be dinner, and this can be a normal dinner for you. Let's say you have your last meal on a Friday night; you won't eat again until Sunday morning. This way, your fasting clock will start around 7:00 p.m., and by 7:00 a.m. the next day you'll be one-third of the way finished.

Throughout the fast keep drinking plenty of water. This will not only keep you hydrated, it will help flush out excess sugar and toxins from your bloodstream and internal organs. If you get tired of water you can switch to black coffee or myriad different types of teas. There are dozens of flavors to try, with or without caffeine: Just don't add sugar or milk.

If you're feeling really run down, or really tired during the fast, don't reflexively reach for food. Instead, try to drink water, go for a walk, get a massage, take a nap, read, whatever you need to do to just blast through this. Whatever you do, don't fall back into your old habits of eating bad carbs.

It's very likely that at some point during or after the fast you'll feel tired, just as I did. This fatigue might take a day or two to set in. The reason for this fatigue is that you have depleted your muscle glycogen stores. Glycogen is your muscles' main source of energy. Knowing this is coming will help you get through it. You also need to know that this feeling will go away on its own, because once you start burning body fat you'll produce ketones, which are another source of energy your muscles and brain can use in place of glycogen and glucose. As you become ketotic, you'll feel re-energized. You may even find that your energy levels will come back to normal or even better than normal, and that's how you will continue to feel as long as you're following this JumpStart program.

When you experience this increased energy, you literally become a fat-burning machine. You've turned your entire metabolism around: Before you were not tapping into your fat stores at all for energy, but now you're tapping almost exclusively into your fat stores for energy. You will start dropping body fat like mad. By the time you get to Week 3 and start the Basic Health Diet, you will begin moving back to making glycogen from glucose and storing it, so that your exercise will be supported by its most efficient energy source.

However, if at any time during the initial fast you feel dizzy, sweaty, or weak, stop the fast immediately. These could all be signs of dehydration or very low blood sugars. If this happens, first drink a couple of glasses of water and see how you feel. If you don't feel better in a few minutes stop your fast and start on the Basic Health Diet.

General Cooking Guidelines

The way you prepare foods significantly affects their nutrient levels. For instance, while many tout the benefits of eating "raw," it turns out that vegetables have higher antioxidant levels when they are heated, as long as you don't boil them, stripping away their valuable nutrients. The best way to maximize their nutrient content is by using a microwave pressure cooker or steamer.

Unless you are a chef and love cooking you need to keep it simple. My experience is that the easier you can make your food preparation the more likely you will incorporate it into your lifestyle now and for the rest of your life. Animal proteins should always be thoroughly cooked, using the smallest amount of additional fats in order to keep the calorie count down.

When you do need to cook with fats, I always stay away from butter and margarine and choose olive oil, but you can also use canola oil: These are both rich in omega-3 fatty acids. Broiling and grilling are the cleanest, best-tasting options that require the least amount of additional fats for the cooking process. Microwaving can be fat-free but often leaves animal proteins feeling rubbery, so it's not my first choice. Baking and sautéing typically require a sauce to keep fish or poultry moist, adding unnecessary calories, fats, or sugar.

When it comes to cooking grains I like to use microwave brown rice that comes in individual packets instead of steaming a whole pot. I season the cooked rice with a little sea salt and fresh-ground pepper, which is a much healthier alternative than chicken broth. Sometimes I make a large pot of quinoa or wild rice that will last a week, making it much easier to portion out and eat when I'm feeling hungry, instead of waiting for it to be fully cooked and snacking on something else in the meantime.

You'll notice that I don't add salt to any of my meals and to just a few of the recipes. However, most of us really don't have to worry about how much salt we eat. Only about 20 percent of men are salt-sensitive. You can tell if you are if you notice that whenever you consume salt you feel bloated. It turns out that the salt is making you retain excess fluid, which leads to an increase in your circulatory volume. This increases the work your heart must perform and can also increase your blood pressure. If you are not salt-sensitive and don't have a family history of hypertension (high blood pressure), you can continue to use salt in your cooking. You can also eat foods that have sodium in them as long as you do so in moderation. However, you need to recognize that most men eat way too much salt. I have found that if you do cut down on salt you will begin to appreciate other flavors in foods a lot more and become less inclined to crave processed foods or fast foods. A better option is adding spices to any of these meals: They have virtually no calories, will add tons of flavor, and best of all contain powerful antioxidants.

Days 2 to 6

Week 1 is going to be the phase that will help you switch from being a "sugar burner" to a "fat burner." For the rest of the first week, you'll be following a diet that is exclusively composed of three high-protein meals a day. Each meal is accompanied by vegetables. This is a great way to transition back into eating and at the same time continuing to drop weight quickly. Space out your meals evenly throughout the day, and finish your last meal no later than 7:00 p.m. whenever possible.

The following lists a variety of suggestions for each meal. They are all perfectly balanced to contain the right protein/carb ratio. Each meal is easy to prepare and requires little beyond what you may need for cooking (i.e., a tablespoon of olive oil when necessary).

You don't have to eat all of the meals listed, but you certainly can try them all. You can even interchange them throughout the day: If you prefer your eggs in the afternoon, or don't eat certain foods, skip over them, but do not replace with foods that are not on this list. This is critical for your success in the first week of the diet. The recipes for some, particularly the shakes, are listed when required.

Breakfast suggestions:

- 5 egg white omelet made with 2 pieces of string cheese and 1 cup fresh spinach

- 1 cup cottage cheese sprinkled with 2 oz chopped almonds and 1 cup of sliced tomatoes

- 1 whey protein shake (see page 186) and 2 tbs peanut butter spread over 2 stalks celery

- 6 oz smoked salmon, spread with 2 tbs whipped cream cheese

- 2 eggs any style and 1 cup plain low-fat Greek yogurt

- 1 casein protein shake (see page 186)

Lunch suggestions:

- Salad: toss 2 cups mixed greens, 1 cup shredded red cabbage, 4 oz (small) chicken breast, ½ cup tomato, ½ cup cucumber, 2 tbs fat-free Italian dressing

- 6 "extra jumbo" shrimp and 8 asparagus spears

- Salad: toss 4 oz canned tuna (packed in water, not oil), 2 cups shredded lettuce, ½ cup tomato, ½ small red onion (chopped), ¼ cup olives, 2 tbs fat-free Italian dressing

- 4 oz lean chopped beef burger and 1 cup steamed broccoli (no bun)

- 4 oz fresh turkey breast and 1 cup string beans

- 4 oz chicken breast and 1 cup fresh spinach

Dinner suggestions:

- 4 oz flounder and 2 cups bok choy

- 4 oz steak, 2 cups kale

- 5 oz mahi mahi, 1 cup string beans, and 1 cup tomatoes

- 5 oz pork chop, 1 cup artichoke hearts

- 4 oz very lean T-bone steak with 2 cups zucchini and 1 cup Brussels sprouts

- 4 oz chicken breast and ¾ cup eggplant

Assess How You Feel

Many of my patients tell me that when they're on a diet for a couple of weeks, all of a sudden they feel bad, both physically and mentally. They report feeling tired, lethargic, weak, and irritable, so much so that many throw in the towel and quit. Some even report having serious cravings for the foods they have been working so hard to avoid. I certainly know what this feels like. But what they don't know, and what other diet books don't really talk about, is that this is the part of the weight-loss process that actually needs to occur. There is a physiological reason for this, and if you know to expect it you're more likely to be able to get past it and ultimately succeed.

After a week or two following a high-protein/low-carb diet it is almost expected that you will be in a crappy mood. I get to a point where I feel just unbelievably exhausted, and am craving bread, or potatoes, or something. It's actually a form of withdrawal: Your body needs to get used to less glycogen and using body fat for your energy needs. If you can tough it through, you'll start producing the ketones we've been talking about, and you will begin to metabolize your body fat. Depending on your current health, previous eating habits, and muscle mass, it may take up to 10 days to achieve a full-blown ketosis state. Then you really start feeling better. Actually, in many cases, you feel more energized than you've ever felt. Your local drugstore may carry a simple urine test (ketosis strips) so that you can determine when you achieve ketosis.

At the end of every week, take your waistline measurements and weigh yourself. If you have been following these instructions carefully you should begin to see some movement on the scale. Remember, belly fat is the hardest to move, so don't be discouraged if you haven't lost a full inch yet. But keep going: You will see results soon.

REAL MEN, REAL MOTIVATION: LETTER FROM MY FRIEND

I owned a restaurant for 28 years. A restaurant's a lot like a car, it only runs by itself downhill. So I was in the restaurant from 9:00 in the morning to 10:00 at night. I never had a moment's peace. Every meal I would just grab a hoagie roll, throw some tomatoes and cheese and some ham on it. I never sat down to eat a meal in 28 years. Eventually my waist got up into the 50s (inches).

Last Christmas my son came home from school and I asked him, "What do you want me to get you for Christmas?" He said, "Dad, I want you to lose weight. That's what I want for me. I want you to lose weight."

I sat down and I just got pissed off. I was 62 years old. Back in the day I was an all-state high school and college football player. I always took care of my body. Even into my mid-30s when I opened the restaurant I was doing fine. But my life took over. You just get so caught up in the things you're doing day-to-day that you start to not take care of yourself. Then I thought about my friend and my doctor, Jeff Life, and I realized that if he could lose the weight and get back into shape, then I could do it. I looked at Jeff in those pictures, and I got Jeff's first and second books. I've seen him on TV. I knew I could do that. If you look at Jeff you're going to be motivated. You look at the picture, a picture doesn't lie. It's right there in front of you.

I followed the program and started using my body fat as energy. I got myself into ketosis three or four days into this. I've been strictly following this diet for eight and a half months. In total I've lost 120 pounds, 22 inches off my waist. But I don't think about this as pounds lost. I think of it as sticks of butter lost. If I lost two pounds, it's like eight more sticks of butter. Right now I've lost 480 sticks of butter. Just imagine 20 sticks of butter side by side across the table, stacked 24 high. That's part of my body that my heart doesn't have to pump blood through.

The most beautiful thing is that I have not had a craving in eight and a half months for anything. I have literally not once put one thing on my lips that shouldn't have been on my lips. I'm talking about ice cream, bread, pasta, pizza. I eat on schedule, on time, rather than on hunger. I'm Italian. Not eating pasta and bread is for me like peeing in the ocean to change the water temperature. It's just unfathomable that you can't even think about me not eating a piece of bread in my hand. But I have not had one craving in eight and a half months. I have not sat down and said, man, I just want a piece of bread, or I want pasta. I've sat down at tables with people eating pizza in front of me, or eating chips, things that are all my weaknesses. I have not felt the need to put one of those things in my mouth. Once your head gets into what you want to do, and you kept those carbs down to next to nothing and you're not living off the insulin being pumped out by your pancreas for your sugar, and you get into ketosis, the diet becomes easy. To be honest, I have not struggled to lose the 120 pounds.

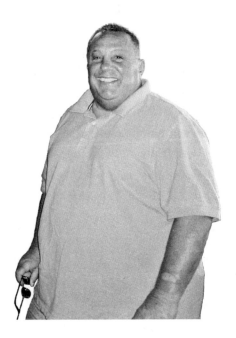

Sal 2012

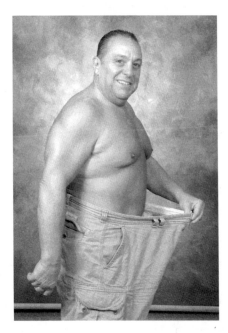

Sal 2013

The day I started I went down to my local YMCA and got on the elliptical.
I did eight minutes. I thought I was going to die. Now I'm doing five miles a day in
30 minutes. Since I started on the 30th of December, I've missed four days at the YMCA
working out. That was Easter Sunday, Memorial Day, Fourth of July, and Labor Day.
Those were the days that it was closed. Now I've got over 50 or 60 people at YMCA
doing the same thing.

As a matter of fact, I put my son's pants on that he wore to high school, and I've
been wearing them around for the last two or three weeks. They're a size 34 pants. He's
a little bit mad at me because he's wearing 36 now. I feel good, I sleep better, I'm eating
wholesome. I feel like I'm 30 years old again.

Right now, I've got about another inch and a half to lose in my waist before I can
fit comfortably into my purple bell bottom pants I wore in college in 1972. When I lose
this extra inch and a half, I'm really going to be sexy.

Sal M.

Week 2: Transition to Increase Meal Frequency

Week 2 features virtually the same food selections as Week 1, but adds a complex carbohydrate every day around lunchtime. This additional nutrient provides a minimal amount of extra calories without disrupting the protein/carbohydrate ratio. It will help you prepare to re-enter the glycogen process so that you will begin to have enough energy for your exercise program. You need to have a glucose store of glycogen in your muscles to match up your performance with your caloric intake.

This week also transitions you from a three-meal-a-day program to one that has four meals: breakfast, lunch, dinner, plus one snack. This will further help you move seamlessly into a five- to six-meal program. The snack can be eaten between breakfast and lunch, or lunch and dinner. Follow the same directions as listed for Week 1, space out your meals evenly throughout the day, and finish your last meal no later than 7:00 p.m. whenever possible.

Breakfast suggestions:

- 5 egg white omelet made with 2 pieces of string cheese and 1 cup fresh spinach

- 1 cup cottage cheese sprinkled with 2 oz chopped almonds and 1 cup of sliced tomatoes

- 1 whey protein shake (see page 186) and 2 tbs peanut butter spread over 2 stalks celery

- 6 oz smoked salmon, spread with 2 tbs whipped cream cheese

- 2 eggs any style and 1 cup plain low-fat Greek yogurt

- 4 slices turkey bacon with 1 egg

- 1 casein protein shake (see page 186)

Lunch suggestions:

- Salad: 2 cups mixed greens, 1 cup shredded red cabbage, 4 oz chicken breast, ½ cup tomato, ½ cup cucumber, ½ cup quinoa (cooked), 2 tbs fat-free Italian dressing

- 6 "extra jumbo" shrimp, 8 asparagus spears, 1 cup cooked wild rice

- 4 oz canned tuna, 2 cups shredded lettuce, ½ cup tomato, ½ small onion, chopped, 2 oz olives, 2 tbs fat-free Italian dressing, 1 slice Ezekiel bread

- 4 oz lean chopped beef burger and 1 cup of steamed broccoli, a cooked yam (sweet potato)

- 4 oz turkey breast and 1 cup string beans, 1 cup cooked wild rice

- 4 oz broiled chicken breast with 1 cup spinach, 1 cup cooked wild rice

- 2 oz nitrate-free turkey jerky and 1 slice of Ezekiel bread, ½ cup cucumber slices

Dinner suggestions:

- 4 oz flounder and 2 cups bok choy

- 4 oz steak and 2 cups kale

- 5 oz mahi mahi, 1 cup string beans, and 1 cup tomatoes

- 5 oz pork chop and 1 cup artichoke hearts

- 4 oz very lean T-bone steak with 2 cups zucchini and 1 cup Brussels sprouts

- 4 oz chicken breast and ¾ cup eggplant

- 4 oz trout, 2 cups cabbage, and ¼ cup roasted red peppers

Snacks:

- 2 hard-boiled eggs

- 2 tbs all-natural peanut butter and celery sticks

- 1 cup low-fat Greek yogurt

- 4 oz broiled chicken breast

- 1 cup of sliced colorful vegetables (any variety)

- ½ oz of any unsalted nut

- Protein shake

- Protein bar (see page 99 for suggestions)

Exercise on the JumpStart Diet Is Limited

While you follow the Jump Start Diet you cannot exercise beyond walking 15 minutes a day. The reason is that this diet is deliberately designed to deplete your glycogen stores to rapidly get you into a fat-burning state. You just won't have the energy to do much in the way of serious exercise.

However, 15 minutes on the treadmill, or a quick walk around the block, is not only a quick way to burn some calories, it really does aid in digestion. In one 2009 study, researchers found that walking has a significant effect on blood sugar after meals. However, researchers found that a walk after dinner led to lower postmeal blood sugar levels in people with type 2 diabetes than either a walk before dinner or no walking at all. Another study, published in *Diabetes Care*, found that in older adults who were overweight and sedentary, walking for 15 minutes shortly after each meal improved daily blood sugar levels to a greater extent than a single 45-minute walk in the morning. This may be because a postmeal walk helps clear glucose from the bloodstream as it is absorbed by the muscles.

Assess How You Feel

By increasing your carbohydrate intake you may begin to feel much better as your body returns to creating more glycogen. Notice how you physically feel eating slightly more often, and having a bit more food every day. Do you feel like you have more energy, or are you still fatigued? Check in with your thoughts about specific foods: Have you had any cravings? And if you did, think about how you handled them, and what can you do better next time. Or, congratulate yourself if you were able to "ride the wave" and get past the craving. Then, check in on your thinking in general: Is your brain fog beginning to lift? Has your attention improved? You may be pleasantly surprised that your concentration has improved, as well as your sleep.

REAL MEN, REAL MOTIVATION: LETTERS FROM MY FANS

Dear Dr. Life,

I was until very recently beginning to think that at 56 I ought to give in to senescence. Your story, reported today in Britain on the BBC, was the kick up the backside I needed. Inspirational. Best wishes,

Paul

The Next Step

After Week 2 move directly to the Basic Health Diet, no matter what your results were. If you loved the fast as much as I did, you can revisit this cycle every eight weeks, where it will jumpstart your weight loss every time.

CHAPTER 8

The Basic Health Diet

Weeks 3 and 4

The meal plans in this chapter represent my recommendations for a basic, healthy diet. It is a low-glycemic, insulin-controlling diet, designed to reduce blood pressure and cardiovascular disease while improving overall health and body composition. In other words, you will continue to lose belly fat by following this eating plan. It focuses on natural, unprocessed foods, with a few packaged foods thrown in for ease.

For the next two weeks, you'll be following a diet that is perfectly balanced between protein, carbohydrates, and healthy fats. You'll be eating five or six smaller meals every day at three- to four-hour intervals. Make sure to finish your last meal no later than 7:00 p.m. whenever possible.

The difference between the Basic Health Diet and the one you were following last week is that instead of each meal's being balanced, I've done the calculations for you for the entire day. By the time you've finished your last meal you will have eaten approximately 1,800 calories comprising more than 150 grams of protein, 300 grams of healthy carbohydrates, and less than 50 grams of fat. Because the entire day is balanced, you don't have the flexibility of swapping one meal for another as you did on the last diet. However, you can repeat any days that you would like. I've provided seven days of meal plans for this diet, which you will follow for the next two weeks. Rotate through the entire menu twice, or repeat any of the full days that you prefer the most.

You can substitute some of my wife Annie's favorite recipes, which are listed in Chapter 11, in order to keep the food choices fresh. These recipes have a perfectly balanced protein/carb/healthy fat ratio, so it won't disrupt the diet. The recipes are coded to show which are appropriate for these next two weeks as well as the next two levels that follow (Fat-Burning and Heart Health). They are designed so that you can prepare more than one serving at a time. You can either share your leftovers or store them for later use.

During these two weeks continue drinking lots of water, tea, and coffee. The recipes for the shakes also appear in Chapter 11. The protein powder in these shakes makes a big impact on the plan, so don't skip these meals. But even I get to a point where I can't drink another shake. When that happens, I'll sometimes add protein powder to my oatmeal in the morning. Heating or cooking the powder unwinds the string of amino acids in the protein molecule and breaks it into smaller pieces. In other words, it starts the digestive process and makes it easier for you to process amino acids and get them into your bloodstream faster, providing energy and boosting your overall metabolism.

You'll also notice that beginning with the Basic Health Diet you will be eating a lot of fruit. I've made sure that all of the fruit suggestions fall into the low-glycemic category. Many low-carb diets avoid fruits, but after Week 2 I embrace them. A 2013 article appearing in the *Journal of American Medicine* supports my thinking. Researcher Dr. David Ludwig, the director of the New Balance Foundation Obesity Prevention Center at Boston Children's Hospital, found that sugars consumed in fruit are not linked to any adverse health effects, no matter how much you eat. His observational studies also showed that increased fruit consumption is tied to lower body weight and a lower risk of obesity-associated diseases. The reason is that colorful fruits contain high levels of antioxidants, healthful nutrients, and fiber. The fiber makes us feel full and provides other metabolic benefits.

Just as with the first two weeks, the meals here are easy to prepare and require little beyond what you may need for cooking. When necessary, the instructions for preparing the meal are listed along with the ingredients.

Poultry and fish are the most popular choices for lean meats that are high in protein, but don't feel that you have to limit yourself to those options. You'll see that a few meal plan days include steak and pork. Lean varieties of both of these options are high in protein and low in fat. Today's pork has a fat content so low that it favorably compares to chicken. The leanest cuts are pork tenderloin, loin chops, and loin roasts. There are also recipes for seafood, particularly shrimp and scallops. Both of these are great options for men, because they contain the right amount of healthy fats and are super easy to prepare.

One of the things I love most about this part of the diet is the addition of my wife Annie's kale soup. The recipe can be found on page 168. Every week she makes a big pot, and we keep it in the fridge so it's ready to reheat. Soup is a great way to get lots of vegetables into your body, especially if you aren't crazy about the way they taste. Soup also fills you up and keeps you satisfied for a long time.

Day 1 Basic Health Diet

MEAL #1

Ingredients: ½ cup quick-cooking steel-cut oats, ½ cup blueberries, 5 egg whites, ½ cup 1% milk

Directions: Combine oats and milk in a large microwave-safe dish. Cook in microwave oven on high for 3 minutes or until oatmeal is thoroughly cooked to the consistency you prefer: More time may be needed. Top with blueberries. In a separate, lightly oiled pan, scramble the egg whites and serve on the side.

MEAL #2

Ingredients: 1 large apple, 1 scoop whey protein powder

Directions: Use the whey powder to make a shake according to the directions on the package. For added flavor, see the recipes in Chapter 11. You can add the apple to the shake (cored and peeled first) or eat separately.

MEAL #3

Ingredients: 4 oz canned tuna (in water, not oil), 2 cups shredded lettuce greens, ½ cup tomato, ½ cup cucumber, ½ small white onion, chopped, ¼ cup olives, 2 tbs fat-free Italian dressing, 1½ cups "Not So Portuguese" kale soup (see recipe on page 168).

Directions: Combine all the ingredients (except for the soup) on a single plate to create a salad. Reheat soup before eating.

MEAL #4

Ingredients: 2 stalks celery, 2 tbs natural reduced-fat peanut butter, 1 large pear

MEAL #5

Ingredients: 4 oz 96% lean beef, 1 yam, 8 asparagus spears, ½ cup red pepper slices
Directions: Broil the beef, bake or microwave the yam. The asparagus and red peppers can be roasted or lightly blanched.

Day 2 Basic Health Diet

- -

MEAL #1

Ingredients: 1 cup low-fat cottage cheese, ½ cup raspberries, ½ cup low-fat granola
Directions: Combine ingredients in a single bowl.

MEAL #2

Ingredients: 1 cup cherries, 2 pieces string cheese

MEAL #3

Ingredients: 6 "extra jumbo"–sized shrimp, 4 tbs salsa, 3 cups mixed greens, ¼ avocado, 1 yam
Directions: Boil the shrimp until firm and pink. Remove shells. Place on a bed of salad greens with the sliced avocado. Use the salsa as a salad dressing. Bake or microwave the yam to serve on the side.

MEAL #4

Ingredients: 1 oz nitrate-free turkey jerky, 1 large pear

MEAL #5

Ingredients: 1 large chicken breast, 20 pine nuts, 1 cup steamed broccoli, 1 cup steamed bok choy, 1 cup cooked wild rice

Directions: Coat the chicken with 1 tbs extra-virgin olive oil and then broil a few minutes on each side until fully cooked (timing will depend on the thickness of the breast). Combine pine nuts and vegetables with cooked rice before eating.

Day 3 Basic Health Diet

MEAL #1
Ingredients: 2 large egg whites, 1 oz 2% shredded cheddar cheese, ½ bell pepper, ½ tomato, ½ small white onion, chopped, 1 large peach
Directions: Stir egg whites together and pour into a lightly greased frying pan over medium heat. Add the cheese, bell pepper, tomatoes, and onions. Pull eggs toward the center until thoroughly cooked. Eat peach separately.

MEAL #2
Ingredients: 2 cups steamed bok choy, sliced, 1 cup cooked quinoa, 1 cup artichoke hearts
Directions: Combine all ingredients for a salad.

MEAL #3
Ingredients: 2 cups chopped kale, 1 tbs sesame seeds, 1 tbs sesame seed oil
Directions: Stir-fry kale in oil and sprinkle with seeds before serving.

MEAL #4
Ingredients: 4 oz turkey breast, 1 cup broccoli, 2 pieces string cheese

MEAL #5
Ingredients: 1 small apple, 1 cup low-fat Greek yogurt

MEAL #6
Ingredients: 4 oz lean top round steak, 2 cups chopped kale, 1 cup cauliflower, 1 yam
Directions: Broil steak for 4 to 6 minutes on each side (timing will depend on the thickness of the meat and how thoroughly cooked you prefer it); steam greens and cauliflower in the microwave for 2 minutes; microwave the yam for an additional 10 minutes.

Day 4 Basic Health Diet

MEAL #1

Ingredients: 1 cup low-fat plain Greek yogurt, ½ cup blueberries, 23 almonds, unsalted
Directions: Combine ingredients in a single bowl.

MEAL #2

Ingredients: 1 peach, 1 oz nitrate-free turkey jerky

MEAL #3

Ingredients: 3 cups mixed greens, 4 oz chicken breast, ½ cup tomato, ½ cup cucumber, 2 tbs fat-free Italian dressing, 1 cup shredded red cabbage, 1 orange or tangerine, sectioned, 1½ cups "Not So Portuguese" kale soup
Directions: Broil or grill the chicken a few minutes on each side until fully cooked (timing will depend on the thickness of the breast). Combine with the rest of the ingredients in a single bowl to create a salad. Serve soup on the side.

MEAL #4

Ingredients: 1 cup cooked wild rice, 2 hard-boiled eggs, 1 cup strawberries

MEAL #5

Ingredients: 4 oz salmon, 1 cup string beans, 1 cup sliced tomatoes, 2 slices Ezekiel bread
Directions: Grill or broil the fish.

Day 5 Basic Health Diet

MEAL #1

Ingredients: 1 scoop whey protein powder, 18 cashews, unsalted, 14 cherries, pits removed
Directions: Combine all the ingredients in a blender to make a shake. Add water as directed on package of whey protein powder.

MEAL #2

Ingredients: 1 tbs natural reduced-fat peanut butter, 1 large apple

Directions: Spread peanut butter on apple slices.

MEAL #3

Ingredients: 1 cup cooked brown basmati rice, 2 tbs extra-virgin olive oil, 6 "extra jumbo"–sized shrimp, 8 asparagus spears, sliced, 1 cup eggplant, cubed

Directions: Toss shrimp, asparagus, and eggplant in olive oil, then grill or broil.

MEAL #4

Ingredients: ¾ cup low-fat cottage cheese, 1 large peach

MEAL #5

Ingredients: 2 cups shredded salad greens, ½ cup garbanzo beans, ½ cup chopped tomato, ½ cup cucumber, ½ small white onion, chopped, ¼ cup olives, 2 tbs fat-free Italian dressing

Directions: Combine all ingredients to create a salad.

MEAL #6

Ingredients: 4 oz broiled pork chop, 1 cup cooked quinoa, 1½ cups chopped kale, ¼ cup mushrooms

Directions: Broil the chop a few minutes on each side until fully cooked (timing will depend on the thickness of the chop and how well-done you prefer it). Steam the kale and mushrooms together in the microwave for 2 minutes and serve over the quinoa.

Day 6 Basic Health Diet

- -

MEAL #1

Ingredients: 3 oz smoked salmon, 1 tbs low-fat whipped cream cheese, 2 slices Ezekiel bread, 1 cup frozen grapes

Directions: Spread cream cheese on bread and top with salmon. Serve grapes on the side.

MEAL #2

Ingredients: 1 large apple, 1 scoop whey protein powder

Directions: Prepare shake with protein powder. See recipes for added flavor in Chapter 11.

MEAL #3

Ingredients: 3 cups mixed greens, 3 oz canned tuna (packed in water), ½ red pepper, ½ small onion, chopped, ¼ cup cilantro, 2 oz black beans, 2 tbs oil and vinegar dressing

Directions: Combine all ingredients to make a filling salad.

MEAL #4

Ingredients: 1 protein bar (see page 99 for suggested brands), 1 large peach

MEAL #5

Ingredients: 4 oz chicken breast, 2 cups cabbage, 2 oz roasted red peppers, ¼ cup spinach, 1 cup wild rice

Directions: Cook chicken breast and slice. Combine remaining ingredients as a salad and top with chicken.

MEAL #6

Ingredients: 1 cup cherries, 1 cup low-fat Greek yogurt

Day 7 Basic Health Diet

MEAL #1

Ingredients: Dr. Life's Protein Pancakes (see page 165 for recipe), ½ cup blueberries

MEAL #2

Ingredients: 1 cup plain low-fat Greek yogurt, ½ cup low-fat granola

MEAL #3

Ingredients: 4 oz orange roughy, 1 yam, 2 cups spinach, 1 cup artichoke hearts

Directions: Broil fish a few minutes on each side until fully cooked (timing will depend on the thickness of the fillet) and microwave the yam for 10 minutes; steam spinach and artichoke hearts in the microwave for no more than 2 minutes and serve together.

MEAL #4

Ingredients: 3 oz low-fat, extra-firm tofu, 1 medium pear

Directions: You can eat firm tofu right out of the package, or if you prefer, you can warm it up in a sauté pan with a tiny drop of olive oil. Heat until slightly browned. Slice the pear and eat together.

MEAL #5

Ingredients: 4 oz very lean T-bone steak, ½ cup cooked quinoa, 2 cups zucchini, 1 cup Brussels sprouts

Directions: Broil or grill steak and zucchini; steam Brussels sprouts.

Assess How You Feel

When you switch to a diet on which you are eating smaller portions more frequently, you probably will begin to feel better both physically and mentally. Physically, you are controlling your blood sugar spikes, because glucose is now being released into your bloodstream in slow and steady increments throughout the day. This alone will make a significant difference in your energy levels. You've also been eating slightly more food than you were allowed during the first two weeks, so you should feel a little fuller at the end of the day. However, it's important for you to realize that you've been consuming approximately the same number of calories that you did in the first two weeks, even though you are eating more frequently. What that means is that once you consistently make the right food choices, you literally can eat more food, and dieting won't feel as if you are depriving yourself or leaving yourself hungry.

Mentally, you may also feel calmer and better able to handle stress. By this point, if you've been really diligent about following the diet, your cravings should have completely subsided. That doesn't mean that you aren't tempted to eat foods that are bad for you: Your body is just not likely to have a physical craving reaction. Check in to see if you were bored with the food choices, or if you liked the structure of a defined eating plan. Did you take advantage of the additional recipes?

Do you feel that you have more energy, or are you still fatigued? Check in on your thinking in general: Is your brain fog beginning to lift? Has your attention improved? You may be pleasantly surprised that your concentration has improved, as well as your sleep.

Begin to Ramp Up Your Exercise

During these two weeks you can increase your daily walk to 30 minutes and try to pick up the pace. If you are walking with a friend or your partner, you should be moving at a pace at which you cannot carry on a conversation. It doesn't matter how far you are going as long as you keep moving.

If you are the competitive type, as I am, look into the Nike+ FuelBand. It works in conjunction with a mobile app so that you can track how active you are throughout the day and measure that in the ways that are important to you. It counts the number of steps that you've taken, calories burned, the distance you've gone, and the time you spent walking. When you wear it all day long, it can show you exactly how active you really are. While it's a little pricey, it's still much cheaper than bypass surgery. Just saying.

REAL MEN, REAL MOTIVATION: LETTERS FROM MY READERS

Dr. Life,

Saw you on *The Doctors* show yesterday. Great publicity for you, your dynamite book. I am on my second reading of your best-selling book. You are a great inspiration to me and for sure every person who reads your book. I'm at the gym first thing in the morning, five days a week. I'm pushing 77 and feel like a young 30-year-old. I have more muscle today than when I was a 20-year-old playing varsity football at Northern Illinois University. At my age I am still putting on muscle in this old man's body. Thanks to you. You continue to inspire us oldies.

Fit for Life,
Bob S.

The Next Step

- -

By this time you should see real progress on the scale. A well-balanced diet like this one should allow you to have lost at least three pounds at this point, and your pants should start feeling a little bit looser. Keep going: The longer you can maintain good eating habits the better your results will be. The foods featured over the next two weeks as you follow the Fat-Burning Diet will further positively affect your metabolism so that you can experience even more fat loss.

CHAPTER 9

The Fat-Burning Diet

Weeks 5 and 6

Over the next two weeks you will be ramping up your efforts to eat cleanly by excluding red meat and dairy fat (such as cheese and milk), the biggest sources of saturated/plaque-building fat, and continuing to follow a low-glycemic eating plan. Eliminating these foods will actually stop the progression of plaque—and in some cases reverse plaque buildup.

While the commercial food industry is already doing a good job of removing trans fats from our food supply, no real effort is being made to rid our diets of saturated fats, which come almost exclusively from animal products. Other popular diets such as the Mediterranean Diet, Atkins, Paleo, and South Beach center on animal fat and low-glycemic carbohydrates, which do not protect your heart health, and as I've said earlier, may actually be damaging to it. To my mind, the combination of low-glycemic carbohydrates and getting less than 10 percent of your calories from fat sets you on a heart-healthy path.

However, the fact that you are giving up red meat and dairy doesn't mean you are skimping on protein: There are a wide variety of animal- and plant-based protein sources here so that you are able to maintain the same ratios between carbs, fats, and healthier protein options. For example, I've become a big fan of quinoa, which tastes like a grain but is really a protein-rich seed that comes from South America. One full serving of quinoa is a cup, contains eight grams of protein, and is a good source of iron and fiber. I've also started sprinkling my salads with shelled hemp seeds. These are tiny, like sesame seeds, but add 10 grams of protein for every three tablespoons with a minimum of additional carbohydrates. Other great seed options that are high in protein are sunflower and pumpkin seeds (with the shells removed) and chia seeds. Chia seeds are exactly the same as what was sprinkled on those crazy gag gifts (remember the ads? *"Ch ch ch chia!"*): They are a very hearty plant that grows like crazy. They are also extremely good for you, containing lots of protein as well as fiber. These seeds turn out to be as healthy for you as nuts, without the excess fat or calories.

I've also replaced the dairy options with soy varieties. While cow's milk has the most calcium and almost double the protein of any other type of milk, the fat content is simply too high for the Fat-Burning Diet. Soy milk is a much better option, because it is plant-based and loaded with antioxidants. Studies have shown that regular intake of soy can significantly reduce the risks of prostate cancer in men. Soy milk is made from ground soybeans and water and is still rich in protein and calcium without any saturated fat. It also scores low in calories. There are all kinds of soy "dairy" products on the market that are useful alternatives for dairy: Over the next two weeks you can try soy yogurt and soy cheese. For example, soy cheese has fewer calories and fat than traditional cheeses and has no saturated fat or cholesterol. I'm not as enamored of almond or rice milk as alternatives. Almond milk contains sweetener and much less protein than either soy or cow's milk. Rice milk is very low in fat and calories, but nutritionally it is even weaker than almond milk.

Finally, I've replaced some of the meat options with vegetarian options, including tofu and seitan. Tofu, also referred to as bean curd, is made by coagulating soy milk and then pressing the resulting curds into soft white blocks. Tofu's consistency ranges from firm to creamy, and it is known to absorb the flavor of anything it is cooked with. Seitan is made from wheat gluten and has a much firmer texture and is actually higher in protein. Seitan has the texture of cooked chicken, making it an ideal replacement in sandwiches or anywhere you would traditionally use meat. And because you are using Ezekiel bread for sandwiches, you can use seitan without disrupting your carb ratio, even though it is wheat-based.

I call this the Fat-Burning Diet because it is designed to guide your body down the fat-burning path while preserving your muscle mass. Like the Basic Health Diet, many of these meals are self-explanatory and require no cooking and little preparation. Others require very rudimentary cooking skills, such as chopping, baking, boiling, or broiling. Most of these meals can be prepared in a microwave oven as well. Just complete the instructions that follow the ingredients list to create a satisfying and easy-to-prepare single dish.

For the next two weeks, you'll continue eating five or six smaller meals every day at three- to four-hour intervals. Make sure to finish your last meal no later than 7:00 p.m. whenever possible. By now your body should be used to eating more frequently. You will notice that your mood is more stable throughout the day, and you have more energy.

Again, I've done the ratio calculations for you for the entire day. By the time you've finished your last meal you will have eaten approximately 1,800 calories comprising more than 150 grams of protein, 300 grams of healthy carbohydrates, and less than 50 grams of fat. Because the entire day is balanced, you don't have the flexibility of swapping one meal for another. However, you can repeat any days that you would like. I've provided seven days of meal plans for this diet, which you will follow for the next two weeks. Rotate through the entire menu twice, or repeat any of the full days that you prefer. Again, each meal is easy to prepare and requires little beyond what you may need for cooking. The vegetables can be eaten to your preference: cooked (preferably steamed) or raw. All of the animal proteins should be thoroughly cooked: Microwaved, broiled, and grilled are the healthiest options, followed by baked and sautéed (which require adding small amounts of fat).

You can substitute some of my wife Annie's favorite recipes, which are listed in Chapter 11, in order to keep the food choices fresh, as long as you skip the ones that include red meat and dairy, or make the suggested substitutions. Follow the codes that show which are appropriate for these next two weeks. These recipes are perfectly balanced regarding their protein/carb/healthy fat ratio, so they won't disrupt the diet.

During these two weeks continue drinking lots of water, tea, and coffee. The recipes for the shakes appear in Chapter 11.

Day 1 Fat-Burning Diet

- -

MEAL #1

Ingredients: 3 oz low-fat extra-firm tofu, ½ small white onion, 1 celery stalk, 1 tbs extra-virgin olive oil, ½ cup blueberries, ½ cup quick-cooking steel-cut oats

Directions: Chop the onion, celery, and tofu and sauté over medium heat. In a separate dish, prepare the oatmeal as directed on the box, replacing equal amounts of boiling water if there was a suggestion to include milk. Top oatmeal with blueberries and eat the two dishes for one filling breakfast.

MEAL #2

Ingredients: 1 nectarine, 2 oz nitrate-free turkey jerky

MEAL #3

Ingredients: 4 oz tilapia, 1 cup "Not So Portuguese" kale soup, ¾ cup cooked brown rice
Directions: Broil or grill the tilapia a few minutes on each side until fully cooked (timing will depend on the thickness of the fillet). Serve with the soup and brown rice.

MEAL #4

Ingredients: 1 scoop whey protein powder, 1 medium apple
Directions: Follow recipes in Chapter 11, using soy products instead of cow's milk or yogurt.

MEAL #5

Ingredients: 5 "extra jumbo" shrimp, 1½ cups bok choy, 1 cup snap peas, 3 baby carrots sliced, 2 tsp low-sodium soy sauce, 1 tbs extra-virgin olive oil
Directions: Combine all of these ingredients into one stir-fry.

Day 2 Fat-Burning Diet

MEAL #1

Ingredients: 1 tbs extra-virgin olive oil, 5 egg whites, ½ cup tomato, diced, 3 tbs shelled hemp seeds, ¼ cup cooked steel-cut oats, ½ cup blueberries, ½ cup soy milk
Directions: Heat a sauté pan with the olive oil. Combine the egg whites, tomato, and hemp seeds in the pan over medium heat and cook. In a separate dish, prepare the oatmeal with the soy milk. Top with blueberries.

MEAL #2

Ingredients: 1½ cups whole strawberries, 1 scoop whey protein powder for shake
Directions: Combine ingredients in a blender, following directions on the package, and replacing dairy with soy alternatives.

MEAL #3

Ingredients: 4 oz grilled chicken breast, 3 cups mixed greens, ½ cup tomato, ½ cup cucumber, ½ bell pepper, 1 oz soy mozzarella, ½ small chopped red onion, ½ cup raspberries, 2 tbs raspberry vinaigrette, 1 slice Ezekiel bread

Directions: Combine all the ingredients except for the bread to create a filling salad.

MEAL #4

Ingredients: 1 cup cooked wild rice, 2 slices soy cheese

MEAL #5

Ingredients: 4 oz grilled ahi tuna, 1 cup cooked quinoa, 1 cup snap peas, 1 cup cauliflower

Directions: Grill or broil the tuna; steam the snap peas and cauliflower.

Day 3 Fat-Burning Diet

MEAL #1

Ingredients: 2 scoops whey protein powder shake, ½ grapefruit

Directions: Follow recipes in Chapter 11 using soy products instead of cow's milk or yogurt.

MEAL #2

Ingredients: ½ cup cubed avocado, ¼ cup tomato, 1 oz nitrate-free turkey jerky

MEAL #3

Ingredients: 4 oz halibut, 1 cup spinach, 1 yam, 1 tbs extra-virgin olive oil

Directions: Broil or grill the halibut a few minutes on each side until fully cooked (timing will depend on the thickness of the fillet), coating in olive oil before cooking. Steam the yam in the microwave for 10 minutes, then steam spinach in the microwave separately, for an additional 2 minutes.

MEAL #4

Ingredients: ½ cup canned adzuki beans, rinsed and drained, 1 medium orange

MEAL #5

Ingredients: 1 cup cooked quinoa sprinkled with 3 tbs shelled hemp seeds, 1½ cups "Not So Portuguese" kale soup

MEAL #6

Ingredients: 4 oz chicken breast, 2 cups shredded bok choy, 1 cup cooked brown rice, 1 cup artichoke hearts

Directions: Broil or grill the chicken a few minutes on each side until fully cooked (timing will depend on the thickness of the breast). Serve on top of the brown rice with the bok choy and the artichoke hearts.

Day 4 Fat-Burning Diet

MEAL #1

Ingredients: 4 large scrambled egg whites, ½ grapefruit

MEAL #2

Ingredients: 1 protein bar (see page 99 for brand suggestions), 1 cup blueberries

MEAL #3

Ingredients: 4 oz turkey breast, 1 cup broccoli, 1½ cups yellow squash

Directions: Grill or broil the turkey breast for 7 to 12 minutes on each side until fully cooked (timing will depend on the thickness of the breast). Steam the broccoli and yellow squash together.

MEAL #4

Ingredients: 1 cup canned black beans, rinsed and drained, ½ small chopped red onion, ½ cup tomato

Directions: Combine all ingredients for a filling snack.

MEAL #5

Ingredients: 4 oz grilled or broiled chicken breast, sliced 1½ cups cabbage, 1 cup cooked wild rice, 1½ cups raw or steamed cauliflower

Directions: Grill or broil the chicken breast for 5 to 7 minutes on each side until fully cooked (timing will depend on the thickness of the breast). Combine all ingredients for a filling salad.

MEAL #6

Ingredients: 1 large apple, 1 scoop whey protein powder

Directions: Follow recipes in Chapter 11, using soy products instead of cow's milk or yogurt.

Day 5 Fat-Burning Diet

- -

MEAL #1

Ingredients: ½ cup dry old-fashioned oatmeal, 6 egg whites

Directions: Prepare oatmeal as directed on the package, substituting water or soy milk for milk. In a separate dish, prepare two hard-boiled eggs, eating only the whites.

MEAL #2

Ingredients: 2 stalks celery, 1 tbs natural reduced-fat peanut butter, 1 large apple

MEAL #3

Ingredients: 6 "extra jumbo"–sized shrimp, diced, ½ small chopped red onion, 2 tbs sweet relish, 2 slices Ezekiel bread, 1 large orange

Directions: Clean the shrimp and boil for 1 to 3 minutes or until the shrimp are pink and opaque. Combine the shrimp with the vegetables to create a light sandwich salad. Serve the orange on the side.

MEAL #4

Ingredients: 1 cup blueberries, 1 cup strawberries, 23 almonds, 1 oz nitrate-free turkey jerky

MEAL #5

Ingredients: 5 oz red snapper, ½ cup sliced zucchini, ½ cup cubed eggplant, 1 yam

Directions: Broil or grill the fish, zucchini, and eggplant for a few minutes on both sides until fully cooked. Bake or microwave the yam.

Day 6 Fat-Burning Diet

MEAL #1

Ingredients: 1 cup unsweetened soy yogurt, 1 cup strawberries, 3 tbs shelled hemp seeds

Directions: Combine all the ingredients.

MEAL #2

Ingredients: 1 oz nitrate-free turkey jerky, 1 cup carrots, 1 cup cucumbers

MEAL #3

Ingredients: ½ cup cooked quinoa, ½ cup roasted red peppers, 2 cups fresh spinach

Directions: Combine all the ingredients for a filling salad.

MEAL #4

Ingredients: 4 oz turkey breast, 1 tbs mustard, 2 slices Ezekiel bread, 1 large orange

MEAL #5

Ingredients: 1½ cups "Not So Portuguese" kale soup, 3 oz seitan, warmed, 1 cup string beans, steamed or raw

MEAL #6

Ingredients: 1 cup cooked brown rice, ½ cup canned black beans, rinsed and drained

Day 7 Fat-Burning Diet

MEAL #1

Ingredients: 2 slices soy cheese, 2 slices Ezekiel bread, ½ cup tomato

Directions: Toast bread with cheese and tomatoes on top for a quick and easy grilled cheese sandwich.

MEAL #2

Ingredients: 1 cup unsweetened soy yogurt, 40 frozen grapes

MEAL #3

Ingredients: 4 oz tuna, canned (packed in water), 2 cups shredded lettuce, ½ cup garbanzo beans, ½ cup cucumber, 3 tbs shelled hemp seeds, 2 tbs fat-free Italian dressing

Directions: Combine all ingredients for a delicious and filling salad.

MEAL #4

Ingredients: 2 scoops whey protein drink, 1 tbs natural reduced-fat peanut butter, 2 stalks celery

Directions: Follow recipes in Chapter 11 using soy products instead of cow's milk or yogurt.

MEAL #5

Ingredients: 4 oz salmon, 1 cup Brussels sprouts, 1½ cups summer squash, 1 cup cooked wild rice

Directions: Grill or broil the fish with the vegetables. Serve over rice.

Assess How You Feel

At the end of six weeks, you will feel energized, leaner, and sexier. It's very possible that your growth hormone levels will have increased, as well as your testosterone. You may be thinking of sex more often. As discussed before, one of the real barometers of health is for you to be having or at least thinking of having sex three times a week. This is an important check-in for any man, especially one who is getting fitter, like yourself.

By this point there should be absolutely no reason for you to feel physically bad or deprived. However, if you feel weak or lethargic, or have a persistent low mood, see your doctor.

Continue Moderate Exercise

You can now increase your walking to up to 60 minutes every day if possible, and definitely four to five times per week. You should be able to pick up the pace more easily and feel more athletic overall. You can begin to set distance goals that should be in the miles category, not blocks. You might even want to join a walking club so that you can change your scenery a bit and socialize with other guys who are making the same good choices that you are.

> ### REAL MEN, REAL MOTIVATION: LETTERS FROM MY READERS
>
> I bought your book, *The Life Plan*, and I think it's awesome. You put together a book that needed to be written. . . . If people would take responsibility for their health, the country would save billions in healthcare costs. And feel like a million bucks to boot. I have [been following] the fat-burning diet for just three weeks. . . . I feel the blanket over my brain is gone. I feel sharper mentally. I feel more limber and stronger.
>
> I'm 54 years old with a 32-inch waist. I didn't want to look like 75 percent of the people I know as I grow older. And you made it a whole lot easier. . . . Thank you, Jeffry S. Life. I beat your drums.
>
> Rory G.

The Next Step

You can stay on the Fat-Burning Diet until you reach your fat-loss goals. This is probably where the additional recipes will come in most handy so that you don't get bored. If you start to plateau and don't see any weight or fat loss, go back and do the JumpStart cycle, and then return to this Fat-Burning Diet. That, and more vigorous exercise, which we'll discuss in Chapter 13, may be all you'll need to see more progress.

Once you reach your goals, you can choose to return to the Basic Health Diet forever. Or, if you prefer the choices on this eating plan, just stay here. Remember, this is not an extremely caloric-deficient plan, and with the right exercise program, it will keep you lean and strong.

If you have been diagnosed with or have a family history of heart or vascular disease, or are experiencing sexual dysfunction connected to circulation issues, you're ready to move to the next level: the Heart Health Diet. This is the one I continue to follow to this day.

CHAPTER 10

The Heart Health Diet

Weeks 7 and 8

The Heart Health Diet is a modified vegan diet that combines low-glycemic eating with a low-fat diet so that you can start reversing blood vessel disease if you have it. This is my most extreme approach. The only good fats allowed are fish oil capsules. Fish and nuts are included, but only in very small amounts.

If you are having problems with your sexual health, this is the diet to follow. And if you have already been diagnosed with a heart condition, have a stent, or have had bypass surgery, high blood pressure, or other vascular problems, you will need to follow the Heart Health Diet as closely as possible forever. Significant research has shown that following this type of vegetarian diet can reverse plaque and vascular disease.

The term "vegetarian" encompasses a wide range of dietary practices, including eating vegetables and no animal products (vegans), eating vegetables, dairy products, and eggs (ovo-lacto vegetarians), or no eggs (lacto vegetarians), and eating vegetables with fish or poultry. A purely vegetarian approach (with less than 10 percent fat) is the only diet shown to reverse heart disease. Research in the last three years has demonstrated that vegetarians not only had more optimized cardiac function but also improved vascular reactivity, lowered blood pressure, balanced blood sugar levels, maintained good cholesterol scores, and achieved trimmer bodies.

Many strict vegans are dangerously low in energy-creating nutrients such as protein, essential amino acids, iron, vitamin B_{12}, calcium, vitamin D, and zinc. Because of this, I strongly recommend that vegetarians, and especially vegans, take great care in planning, selecting, and preparing nutritious meals to make sure they are getting adequate amounts of essential nutrients.

Each meal on the Heart Health Diet consists of two portions of carbohydrate and one portion of protein. If you attempt to boost your protein content by mixing two high-carbohydrate, moderate-protein sources (such as beans and rice) in one meal you will be eating more than one portion of carbohydrate and less than one portion of protein. This can result in fluctuating blood sugar levels and increased insulin secretion, which can increase fat storage, decrease fat burning, and heighten hunger cravings.

When you are following the Heart Health Diet you will be having five or six meals a day at three- to four-hour intervals. The same rules apply for this diet as applied for the earlier levels. Continue to drink plenty of water, coffee, and teas.

Day 1 Heart Health Diet

MEAL #1
Ingredients: Dr. Life's Protein Pancakes
Directions: See recipe on page 165.

MEAL #2
Ingredients: 2 stalks celery, 10 baby carrots, 2 scoops whey protein powder, 1 large pear
Directions: Follow recipes in Chapter 11, using soy products instead of cow's milk or yogurt.

MEAL #3
Ingredients: ½ cup hummus, 1 cup sliced cucumbers, 2 slices Ezekiel bread, 40 frozen grapes
Directions: Generously spread hummus on bread slices and top with cucumber. Serve the frozen grapes on the side.

MEAL #4

Ingredients: 3 cups mixed greens, ½ cup tomato, ½ bell pepper, 1 oz soy mozzarella cheese, ½ small chopped red onion, ½ cup raspberries, 2 tbs raspberry vinaigrette, 3 tbs shelled hemp seeds

Directions: Combine these ingredients to make a hearty salad.

MEAL #5

Ingredients: 6 oz seitan, sliced, 1½ cups bok choy, chopped, 1 cup snap peas, 6 baby carrots, sliced, 2 tsp low-sodium soy sauce, 1 tsp extra-virgin olive oil.

Directions: Combine all ingredients as one stir-fry.

MEAL #6

Ingredients: 2 scoops whey protein powder, 1 large apple

Directions: Follow recipes in Chapter 11, using soy products instead of cow's milk or yogurt.

Day 2 Heart Health Diet

MEAL #1

Ingredients: 1 cup egg whites, ½ cup tomato, ½ small chopped red onion, 1 tbs cilantro, ¼ cup cooked steel-cut oats, ½ cup blueberries, soy milk

Directions: Combine the egg whites, tomato, onions, and cilantro in a sauté pan over medium heat and cook. In a separate dish, prepare the oatmeal with soy milk to your desired consistency. Top with blueberries.

MEAL #2

Ingredients: Protein bar (see page 99 for suggested brands), 1 cup strawberries

MEAL #3

Ingredients: 5 oz low-fat tofu, 1 tbs extra-virgin olive oil, 1 tbs garlic, ¼ cup roasted red peppers, 1 medium apple

Directions: Sauté the tofu with the garlic and red peppers until fully cooked.

MEAL #4

Ingredients: 1½ cups "Not So Portuguese" kale soup, ¾ cup cooked brown rice, 6 oz seitan, sliced

Directions: Place the seitan in a frying pan and season with ½ teaspoon of dried oregano and salt and pepper to taste. Sauté the seitan until it's heated through and you see a little bit of crust forming on the slices. Serve over the brown rice and with the soup.

MEAL #5

Ingredients: 6 hard-boiled egg whites, ¼ cup tomato, ½ red pepper

MEAL #6

Ingredients: ½ cup adzuki beans, 1 cup kale, 1 cup shredded red cabbage, 2 tsp low-fat vinaigrette dressing

Directions: Combine all the ingredients into a healthy salad.

Day 3 Heart Health Diet

MEAL #1

Ingredients: 2 scoops whey protein powder, 1 pear

Directions: Follow recipes in Chapter 11, using soy products instead of cow's milk or yogurt.

MEAL #2

Ingredients: 1 slice Ezekiel bread, ½ avocado, ¼ cup tomato, 6 oz seitan

MEAL #3

Ingredients: 1 cup spinach, 1 yam, baked or microwaved, ½ cup canned white beans, drained and rinsed, ½ small chopped white onion, 1 tsp soy sauce

Directions: Combine these ingredients to create a filling salad.

MEAL #4

Ingredients: 4 hard-boiled egg whites, 3 stalks celery

MEAL #5

Ingredients: 2 cups shredded bok choy, 1 cup artichoke hearts, ¼ cup sundried tomatoes, ½ cup adzuki beans, 1 cup cooked quinoa

Directions: Warm the vegetables and beans together like a stir-fry and serve over a bed of quinoa.

Day 4 Heart Health Diet

MEAL #1

Ingredients: ¼ cup steel-cut oats, 3 egg whites, 1 cup blueberries, ¾ cup boiling water

Directions: Combine the oats and water and cook until your desired consistency is reached. Top with blueberries. In a lightly greased separate pan, scramble the egg whites.

MEAL #2

Ingredients: 3 stalks celery, ¼ cup hummus, 1 scoop whey protein powder

Directions: Spread hummus over celery; prepare shake per packaged instructions, replacing liquids with soy milk or water.

MEAL #3

Ingredients: 1½ cups "Not So Portuguese" kale soup, 3 oz seitan, sliced, 1 small peach

Directions: Place the seitan in a frying pan and season with ½ teaspoon of dried oregano and salt and pepper to taste. Sauté the seitan until it's heated through and you see a little bit of crust forming on the slices. Serve over the brown rice and with the soup and peach.

MEAL #4

Ingredients: 1 cup canned black beans, rinsed and drained, ½ small chopped red onion, ½ cup chopped tomato, 2 cups chopped kale, 1 tbs extra-virgin olive oil.

Directions: Combine these ingredients in a large sauté pan and cook until the kale is wilted.

MEAL # 5

Ingredients: 1¼ cups cooked wild rice, 1½ cups broccoli florets

MEAL #6

Ingredients: 3 cups chopped salad greens, ½ cup chopped tomato, ½ cup cucumber, 3 tbs shelled hemp seeds, 4 hard-boiled egg whites, ½ cup blueberries
Directions: Combine all ingredients for a hearty salad.

Day 5 Heart Health Diet

MEAL #1

Ingredients: 6 egg whites, 2 slices soy cheese, ½ red pepper, sliced
Directions: Create an omelet with these ingredients.

MEAL #2

Ingredients: 2 stalks celery, 1 medium apple, 2 scoops whey protein powder
Directions: Follow recipes in Chapter 11, using soy products instead of cow's milk or yogurt.

MEAL #3

Ingredients: 2 slices Ezekiel bread, 3 oz smoked salmon, 1 tomato, sliced

MEAL #4

Ingredients: ½ small chopped red onion, 2 tbs sweet relish, ¼ cup cucumber, diced, ½ cup bean sprouts, ½ cup edamame (boiled soybeans, pods removed)
Directions: Combine all the ingredients to make a filling salad.

MEAL #5

Ingredients: 1 scoop whey protein powder
Directions: Follow a shake recipe in Chapter 11 that includes some nuts.

MEAL #6

Ingredients: 1 Portobello mushroom, 8 asparagus spears, ½ cup sliced zucchini, ½ cup sliced eggplant, 1 yam, 2 tbs extra-virgin olive oil

Directions: Coat all the vegetables lightly with the oil, then grill or broil, except for the yam, which can be microwaved.

Day 6 Heart Health Diet

- -

MEAL #1

Ingredients: 1 tsp extra-virgin olive oil, 6 egg whites, 1 cup spinach, ¼ cup tomato, 1 medium peach

Directions: In a heated skillet, heat the olive oil and then add in the egg whites, spinach, and tomato to create an omelet.

MEAL #2

Ingredients: 1 cup carrots, 1 cup snap peas, ¼ cup low-fat ranch dressing for dipping

MEAL #3

Ingredients: 1¼ cups "Not So Portuguese" kale soup

MEAL #4

Ingredients: 1 cup cooked quinoa, 2 cups shredded bok choy, 1 cup artichoke hearts, 1 oz sundried tomatoes

Directions: Combine all ingredients.

MEAL #5

Ingredients: 1 cup cubed butternut squash, 8 asparagus spears, ¾ cup white beans, drained and rinsed

Directions: Microwave the squash first, then the asparagus spears. Eat both alongside the beans.

MEAL #6

Ingredients: 3 cups mixed greens, 1 cup shredded red cabbage, ½ cup tomato, ½ cup cucumber, 2 tbs fat-free Italian dressing, 4 hard-boiled egg whites

Directions: Combine all ingredients for a filling salad.

Day 7 Heart Health Diet

MEAL #1

Ingredients: ½ cup steel-cut oats, ½ cup blueberries, 3 tbs shelled hemp seeds

Directions: Combine oatmeal and water in a microwave-safe dish and cook on high for 3 minutes until the desired consistency is met. Top with blueberries and hemp seeds.

MEAL #2

Ingredients: 2 scoops whey protein powder, 1 cup cherries

Directions: Follow recipes in Chapter 11, using soy products instead of cow's milk or yogurt.

MEAL #3

Ingredients: 2 cups shredded lettuce, ½ cup garbanzo beans, ½ cup chopped tomato, ½ cup cucumber, ½ small chopped red onion, 2 tbs fat-free Italian dressing

Directions: Combine all the ingredients for a filling salad.

MEAL #4

Ingredients: 2 tbs natural reduced-fat peanut butter, 1 slice Ezekiel bread, 1 cup grapes

MEAL #5

Ingredients: 1 cup black-eyed peas, drained and rinsed, ½ small chopped yellow onion, ¼ cup green pepper, 1½ cups summer squash, 1 cup cooked wild rice

Directions: Combine all the vegetables in a sauté pan and cook until softened. Serve over the rice.

Assess How You Feel

For the first two weeks on this diet you can continue your walking for up to 60 minutes every day if possible, and definitely four to five times per week. Your exercise tolerance should be steadily improving. But you are not going to notice improved heart health until you see your cardiologist. In eight weeks, I would expect that your performance on an exercise stress test will be significantly improved, along with marked improvements in your blood tests, including your cholesterol panel and biomarkers for vascular inflammation.

You can stay on the Heart Health Diet forever, even if you lose all the belly fat you want and see positive testing results with your cardiologist. This is probably where the additional recipes will come in most handy, so that you don't get bored. If you start to plateau and don't see any weight or fat loss, go back and do the fast days of the JumpStart cycle, then come right back and follow the meal plans on this Heart Health Diet. That, and more vigorous exercise, which we'll discuss in Chapter 13, may be all you'll need to see more progress.

CHAPTER 11

Additional Recipes

- -

Healthy eating is possible—no matter how busy you are. The meal plans in the previous chapters are really all you need to get through the first eight weeks of the program. But the Life Plan Diet is a lifestyle, not a quick fix. These recipes help keep you on track once you've accomplished your goals, or provide ways to easily change up the diet so you don't get bored and tempted to eat something you should be avoiding.

My wife, Annie, has made dieting effortless for me. She has revolutionized my ability to stay on track with my nutrition program. If you start following her lead you will never find yourself without healthy food. The secret to her success, and mine, is that she cooks a large batch of everything she makes, and then portions it out and freezes the portions. Then, all I have to do is go into the freezer, and my meals are ready for me to reheat just before I eat. Annie prepares my "protein packs" once a week. I keep some at home and take several to work with me so I never have to think about what I need to eat, or if the foods I need are available.

I also make frozen individual servings of vegetables, which can be microwaved quickly, creating a completely balanced meal: 1 bag of protein, 1 bag of low-glycemic carb (yams, wild rice, or brown rice), and a serving of healthy vegetables.

In order to do this, all you'll need is a food vacuum sealer. Then, choose among Annie's recipes and multiply the yield so that you can make six servings at a time. This way you'll know that you have at least one meal ready to go—that you really enjoy—when you begin the Basic Health Diet. Remember, the whole trick to dieting is to be able to maintain good habits and not fall back into old traps. The better prepared you are, the less likely that this will happen.

Annie's Recipes

These forty meals are all protein-based and can be used on any of the diets. The following notations indicate the diet plan that applies to each: Basic Health Diet (BHD); Fat-Burning Diet (FBD); and Heart Health Diet (HHD). All recipes can be multiplied if you want to prepare your food ahead, or if you are entertaining a friend. Any can be served with a yam, a cup of green vegetables, or a cup of brown rice, wild rice, or quinoa.

For the purposes of following the Life Plan Diet it really doesn't matter when you eat these meals. They are delicious and easy to prepare, especially if you make them ahead of time. Even the breakfast options can be eaten throughout the day: A great-tasting omelet makes a delicious high-protein/low-fat meal any time.

HIGH-POWERED OATMEAL (BHD, FBD, HHD)

Serves 1

Ingredients:
- ½ cup steel-cut oats
- 2 cups water
- 2 scoops whey protein powder (40 g)
- ½ cup fresh blueberries

Directions: In a 2-quart saucepan, bring water to boil. Stir in oats, cover, and reduce heat to low. Simmer slowly and stir often until oats are desired thickness (approx. 15 minutes). Remove from heat. Stir in protein powder and berries and serve.

CREAMY BREAKFAST CRUNCH (BHD, FBD, HHD)

Serves 1

Ingredients:

- 1 cup low-fat Greek yogurt or low-fat cottage cheese (substitute soy yogurt for FBD and HHD)
- ½ cup low-fat granola
- ½ cup fresh or frozen berries (your choice: blueberries, strawberries, raspberries, blackberries)

Directions: Combine all three ingredients into one bowl and serve immediately.

VEGAN BREAKFAST SKILLET (BHD, FBD, HHD)

This is a perfect breakfast for two, but if you are eating by yourself, save half for tomorrow or for a snack later in the day. This dish can be refrigerated and eaten at room temperature.

Serves 2

Ingredients:

- ½ tbs olive oil
- ¼ medium white onion, chopped
- ½ red bell pepper, chopped
- 3 ounces vegan sausage links, cut into ¼-inch slices
- ½ pound extra-firm tofu, drained, pressed, and cut into ½-inch dice
- 6 oz spinach, chopped
- 1 clove garlic, minced
- Juice of ½ lemon
- ½ tsp dried basil
- ½ tsp dried parsley
- ½ tsp dried thyme
- ¼ tsp turmeric
- ½ tsp salt
- Pinch ground cayenne

Directions: Heat olive oil in a large skillet over medium-high heat. Add the onion and cook for 2 minutes. Add the red pepper and veggie sausage links and cook 2 minutes, or until the pepper starts to soften and the sausage begins to brown. Add the tofu, spinach, and garlic. Cook, stirring, for 5 minutes, or until the tofu begins to turn golden. Add the lemon juice, herbs, salt, and cayenne. Cook for 10 minutes to allow the flavors to blend. If the mixture is dry, add a splash of water.

POACHED EGG WITH SMOKED SALMON (BHD, FBD)

I like to make these eggs for breakfast or lunch. They are perfect for this diet because they do not require any added fat for cooking, and they make a great alternative to hard-boiled eggs. Tip: A poaching pot is much easier to clean if it's still warm from cooking.

Serves 1

Ingredients:

1 large egg

Distilled white vinegar

⅛ lb smoked salmon

Cucumber slices

Directions: Break the egg into a small bowl. Fill a large, deep saucepan with at least 3 inches of water. Add 1 tsp of vinegar per each cup of water in the saucepan. Bring to a boil. Reduce to a gentle simmer: The water should be steaming and small bubbles should come up from the bottom of the pan. Submerging the lip of each bowl in the simmering water, gently add the egg. Cook for 4 minutes for a soft set, 5 minutes for medium, and 8 minutes for a hard set. Using a slotted spoon, transfer the egg to a clean dish towel to drain for a minute. Layer the salmon on a plate and place the egg on top before serving. Garnish with cucumber slices.

EGG WHITE OMELET WITH FRESH HERBS (BHD, FBD, HHD)

Ingredients:

4 egg whites with 2 tbs water

1 cup chopped fresh spinach leaves

½ bunch fresh parsley (½ cup)

1 tbs fresh basil, chopped

4 tsp chopped green onion

2 tsp chopped chives

1 tsp fresh chopped dill

Directions: Combine all herbs and spinach in bowl, then mix. Beat egg whites and water until fluffy. Spray skillet with nonstick cooking spray and heat over medium-low heat. Add herb mixture to egg whites and very lightly stir. Pour mixture into skillet and cover. Cook slowly until the egg is almost set. With rubber spatula, fold omelet in half and cook an additional minute. Serve immediately.

DR. LIFE'S PROTEIN PANCAKES (BHD, FBD, HHD)

Ingredients:

½ cup natural oatmeal

1 cup egg whites

Directions: Mix above in blender, then fry in pan with nonfat spray.

QUICK SALMON SALAD (BHD, FBD)

Prepare and freeze into 6 portions. When you are ready to eat, microwave for less than a minute or let it thaw on the counter for about an hour.

Serves 6

Ingredients:

2 lb fresh salmon fillet

2 cups water

1 medium white onion

½ cup celery

½ cup fresh parsley

½ cup fresh dill

Juice from one lemon

Directions: Finely chop onion, celery, parsley, and dill, then mix together in a large bowl. Set aside. Lightly wash the fish. Fill a large, deep skillet with at least 4 inches of water. Add 1 tsp of vinegar per each cup of water in the saucepan. Bring to a boil. Reduce to a gentle simmer: The water should be steaming and small bubbles should come up from the bottom of the pan. Add fish and poach for about 6 to 10 minutes or until fish flakes easily. Remove from heat and drain. Allow fish to cool for about 10 minutes. Afterward, lightly flake the fish with a fork and toss gently with onion mixture. Squeeze lemon juice on top to taste.

ANY MEAT MEATLOAF (ANY MEAT, BHD; IF USING TURKEY OR PORK, FBD)

Serves 4

Ingredients:

- 1 lb lean chopped meat (beef, turkey, pork, or lamb)
- 1 egg white
- 1 red onion, chopped
- 1 red pepper, chopped
- 1 chopped garlic clove
- ¼ cup ground almonds
- 1 tbs oregano
- 1 tbs basil
- 1 tbs thyme

Directions: Preheat oven to 350. Mix all of the ingredients in a bowl. Coat a loaf pan lightly with olive oil. Pour mixture into the loaf pan. Cook in oven for 45 to 55 minutes or until thoroughly cooked.

FRESH MUSHROOM SALAD (BHD, FBD, HHD)

Serves 2

Ingredients:

- 16 oz fresh white mushrooms
- 1 cup freshly chopped parsley
- 1 small onion, minced
- ¼ cup extra-virgin olive oil
- Juice from 1 lemon
- 2 cups mixed greens
- ½ cup sunflower seeds

Directions: Wash mushrooms, trim stems, and slice. Place in a large mixing bowl. Coarsely chop fresh parsley and mix with mushrooms. Add minced onion. Whisk the olive oil and lemon juice together and drizzle over mushrooms, then stir to cover completely. Add fresh ground pepper to taste. Place on top of mixed greens, sprinkle with sunflower seeds, and serve.

OPEN-FACED VEGGIE SANDWICH (BHD, FBD, HHD)

Serves 1

Ingredients:

- 2 slices Ezekiel bread, toasted
- ½ cucumber, sliced lengthwise
- ½ fresh tomato, sliced
- ½ cup spinach leaves
- ¼ cup canned black beans
- ¼ cup carrot, grated
- 1 tbs olive oil mayonnaise
- Dash of lemon juice

Directions: Mash black beans and lemon juice together. Blend in mayonnaise. Spread bean mixture on each slice of toasted Ezekiel bread. Top with cucumber slices, tomato, spinach leaves, sprouts, and carrots.

MAZATLAN SHRIMP WITH SALSA (BHD, FBD)

Serves 8

Ingredients:

- 2 cups diced fresh tomatoes
- 1 cup chopped red bell pepper
- 1 cup chopped fresh cilantro
- ¼ cup diced onion
- 3 lbs fresh shrimp
- 1 tbs olive oil
- Sea salt and pepper to taste

Directions: In a large bowl, mix together the diced tomatoes, chopped peppers, diced onion, and chopped cilantro. Season lightly with sea salt and black pepper. Let stand in refrigerator. Peel and devein the shrimp. Put olive oil in a large skillet and heat slightly over medium heat. Add shrimp all at once and cook until shrimp are just pink. Spoon salsa mixture over shrimp and serve.

ANNIE'S STUFFED TOMATOES (BHD, FBD, HHD)

Replace chicken with equal amount of diced tofu or seitan for HHD.

Serves 2

Ingredients:

- ¼ cup extra-virgin olive oil
- 1 tbs deli style mustard
- Juice from 1 lemon
- 2 large tomatoes, ripe, firm
- 1 tbs minced onion
- ¼ cup diced celery
- ¼ cup chopped almonds
- 3 tbs chopped fresh parsley
- 8 oz grilled chicken breast, tofu, or seitan, chopped
- Fresh-ground pepper to taste

Directions: Combine olive oil, mustard, and lemon juice together to make a dressing and set aside. Cut the tops from the tomatoes and spoon out the flesh and seeds and discard. In a separate mixing bowl, combine chicken, onion, celery, almonds, and 2 tbs of the parsley. Add the dressing and mix well. Fill each hollowed tomato with the mixture and place on platter. Garnish the tops with the remaining 1 tbs of chopped parsley, ground pepper, and serve.

"NOT SO PORTUGUESE" KALE SOUP (BHD, FBD, HHD)

One of my favorite New England dishes is Portuguese kale soup—but it's high in fat. Try my tasty, healthier version. This recipe will make a large batch that you'll have for a week that you can keep in the refrigerator.

Ingredients:

- 2 large (48 oz) cans of 100% fat-free, low-sodium beef broth (use vegetable broth for HHD)
- 1 large yellow onion (chopped)
- 4 to 6 cloves fresh garlic, minced
- 1½ teaspoons crushed red pepper
- 2 cans cannellini beans (rinsed/drained)
- 1 to 2 lbs fresh kale (stems removed/cut)
- Black pepper and/or paprika to taste

Directions: In a large soup kettle, sauté onions in ¼ cup of the broth. Add the remaining broth, red pepper, and garlic. Add the beans and kale, bring to a boil, then stir and lower the heat. Cook just long enough till the kale is tender, about 3 to 4 minutes.

SPICY GRILLED SUMMER VEGETABLES (BHD, FBD, HHD)

Serves 1

Ingredients:

- 1 large zucchini (washed/cut in ¼-inch diagonal slices)
- 1 large yellow summer squash (washed/cut in ¼-inch diagonal slices)
- 1 lb fresh asparagus (diagonally cut into 2-inch pieces)
- 1 bunch fresh basil
- Medium red onion (thinly sliced)
- Olive oil spray
- Crushed red pepper flakes
- 3 tbs shelled hemp seeds

Directions: Warm grill or frying pan to medium heat. Mix veggies together and give them a spritz of extra-virgin olive oil spray. Sprinkle with crushed red pepper flakes to taste. Add fresh basil leaves (whole). Place all ingredients in a nonstick grill wok, or the frying pan, and cook for 15 minutes, stirring often until tender. Sprinkle with hemp seeds before serving.

LEMONY DILL CHICKEN BREAST (BHD, FBD)

Substitute seitan for chicken for HHD.

Serves 4

Ingredients:

- 4 5-oz chicken breasts (boneless/skinless)
- 1 lemon (cut in half)
- 1 tsp paprika
- 8 small sprigs of fresh dill
- 4 tbs capers, rinsed (to reduce sodium)

Directions: Rinse and tenderize chicken breasts. Sprinkle with paprika and squeeze juice from ½ lemon over breasts. Place breasts on aluminum foil. Broil 6 to 8 minutes or until lightly browned. Flip breasts and broil an additional 6 to 8 minutes until lightly browned. Remove from broiler. On each breast, place a few sprigs of fresh dill weed. Next, place 2 or 3 very thin slices of lemon on top of the dill, and 1 tbs of capers on top of that. Return and broil an additional 1 to 2 minutes.

BLACK PEPPER SALMON (BHD, FBD, HHD)

Servings: 6

Ingredients:

2½ lbs fresh salmon fillets

2 red bell peppers, diced

1 medium yellow onion, diced

Marinade:

¼ cup extra-virgin olive oil

¼ cup fresh-ground black peppercorns

3 cloves garlic

Juice from ½ lemon

Directions: Mix olive oil, garlic, pepper, and lemon juice to form a marinade. Place the salmon in a one-gallon-size Ziploc bag and pour marinade over fish. Close tightly and marinate in refrigerator for 1 hour. Meanwhile, mix peppers and onions in bowl and set aside. Preheat oven to 425°F. Place marinated salmon on baking sheet or aluminum foil along with peppers and onions. Bake for 20 minutes or until salmon easily flakes with fork and peppers are just tender. Remove from oven. Divide peppers/onions into 6 portions and serve with fish.

NOT SO NAKED CHICKEN (BHD, FBD)

Substitute seitan for chicken for HHD.

Serves 6

Ingredients:

6 5-oz boneless, skinless chicken breasts

1 lemon

2 cloves garlic

½ tsp rosemary

½ tsp thyme

½ tsp oregano

¼ tsp red chili pepper flakes

¼ tsp paprika

1 tsp extra-virgin olive oil

Directions: Preheat oven to 350°F. Rub the olive oil all over the chicken and place it in a roasting pan with a lid. Rub the garlic gingerly over the chicken. Cut a lemon in half and squeeze the juice over the chicken. Mix together the rosemary, thyme, oregano, red chili pepper, and paprika. Sprinkle the mixture over the chicken and cover the pan with lid or aluminum foil. Roast for approximately 45 minutes.

QUINOA BULGUR TABBOULEH SALAD (BHD, FBD, HHD)

Serves 4

Ingredients:

½ cup quinoa

½ cup bulgur wheat

2 cups water

Salt to taste

1 medium-size ripe tomato, seeded and chopped

¼ cup minced red onion

½ cup canned black beans, rinsed and drained

½ cup fresh parsley, minced

3 tbs chopped mint leaves

⅓ cup extra-virgin olive oil

2 tbs fresh lemon juice

Freshly ground black pepper to taste

Directions: Wash the quinoa thoroughly, then rinse and drain. Bring the water to a boil in a medium-size saucepan. Add salt, bulgur, and quinoa. Reduce the heat to low, cover, and simmer until all the water is absorbed, about 15 minutes. Place the grains in a large serving bowl and set aside to cool. Add the tomatoes, onion, beans, parsley, and mint. In a separate bowl, whisk together the olive oil, lemon juice, and salt and pepper until blended. Pour the dressing over the salad and toss well to combine. Cover and refrigerate for at least 1 hour before serving. Serve chilled.

TURKEY STIR-FRY (BHD, FBD)

Substitute seitan for turkey for HHD.

Serves 4

Ingredients:

2 tsp olive oil

1 lb turkey tenderloin, cut into thin strips

1 cup fat-free vegetable broth

4 garlic cloves, minced

¼ tsp crushed red pepper flakes

¼ tsp salt

1 red bell pepper, cut into thin strips

1 cup fresh broccoli florets

1 cup fresh cauliflower florets

2 tbs soy sauce

Directions: Place a large nonstick skillet over medium-high heat until hot. Add 1 tsp oil to pan, and tilt to coat evenly. Add turkey, and stir-fry 5 minutes or until turkey is no longer pink in center. Remove turkey and set aside. Combine broth and garlic, red pepper flakes, and salt. Set aside. Add remaining 1 tsp oil to pan; add pepper strips, broccoli, and cauliflower; stir-fry 1 minute. Increase heat to high. Stir broth mixture and add to pan with soy sauce, turkey, and any accumulated juices. Bring to a boil; cook 1 to 2 minutes or until slightly thickened.

SEITAN TAGINE (BHD, FBD, HHD)

Serves 4

Ingredients:

1 tsp cumin seeds

1 tsp caraway seeds

1 tsp coriander seeds

½ tsp paprika

½ tsp black peppercorns

1 (1-inch) piece cinnamon stick

2 tsp olive oil

2 cups finely chopped onion

¾ cup finely chopped carrots

½ cup finely chopped celery

½ tsp sea salt

2 garlic cloves, peeled

2 cups (½-inch) cubed, peeled sweet potato

2 cups chopped green cabbage

1½ cups water

1 cup finely chopped tomato

1 tbs fresh lemon juice

⅔ cup water

6 tbs fresh lemon juice

⅓ cup finely chopped parsley

2 tsp ground cumin

2 tsp paprika

½ tsp sea salt

½ tsp ground red pepper

4 garlic cloves, minced

1 lb seitan, cut into ½-inch cubes

Directions: Preheat oven to 350°F. To prepare the tagine, combine the first 6 ingredients in a spice or coffee grinder; process until finely ground. Heat oil in a large sauté pan over medium heat. Add onion, carrot, celery, ½ tsp salt, and 2 peeled garlic cloves; cook 5 minutes, stirring occasionally. Cover, reduce heat to low, and cook 20 minutes. Stir in spice mixture, sweet potato, cabbage, water, and tomato; bring to a boil. Reduce heat; simmer, uncovered, 30 minutes or until thick. Stir in lemon juice and set aside. Combine ⅔ cup water with all remaining ingredients in a large bowl and toss well to coat. Arrange the mixture in a single layer in an 11-by-7-inch baking dish. Cover with foil. Bake at 350° for 35 minutes. Uncover and bake an additional 5 minutes or until liquid is absorbed. Serve over tagine vegetables.

STEAMED TILAPIA FILLET (BHD, FBD, HHD)

Serves 1

Ingredients:

1 (6-oz) tilapia fillet

1 tsp fat-free mayonnaise

Juice from fresh lemon

2 sprigs of fresh dill per fillet

Fresh-ground pepper to taste

Directions: Place 3 inches of water in bottom of steamer pot. Place fillet in top steamer pan. With a pastry brush, spread mayonnaise over fillets. Squeeze lemon juice over each, garnishing with sprig of fresh dill. Grind fresh pepper to taste. Place lid on pan and heat on high until water boils and heavy steam begins. Turn heat to medium and steam for 20 minutes or until fish flakes easily.

SQUASH ITALIANO (BHD, FBD, HHD)

Serves 6

Ingredients:

1 tbs extra-virgin olive oil

12 fresh basil leaves, finely chopped

2 sprigs fresh thyme, finely chopped

2 sprigs fresh oregano, finely chopped

1 clove garlic, crushed

2 medium-large zucchini

2 medium-large yellow squash

½ cup sundried tomatoes

½ cup chia seeds

Directions: In small bowl, combine olive oil with freshly chopped herbs and garlic. Set aside. Bring 2 cups water to boil. Wash and slice zucchini and squash into ½-inch-thick slices and place in top of steamer over the boiling water. Add sundried tomatoes. Keep steamer above water level. Cover tightly with lid and steam for 5 minutes. Remove from heat and allow to stand for one additional minute. Transfer vegetables to a large bowl and toss with olive oil/herb mixture. Sprinkle with chia seeds before serving.

STEAMED CURRIED CHICKEN (BHD, FBD)

Substitute seitan for chicken for HHD.

Serves 4

Ingredients:

- 4 whole 4-oz boneless, skinless chicken breasts
- 3 tsp madras curry powder
- 2 tsp dried dill
- 2 large carrots, diagonally sliced into ½-inch slices
- 2 yams, skin removed, cut into 1-inch-thick cubes.
- 2 medium-sized yellow squash, diagonally cut into ½-inch slices
- 2 medium-sized zucchini, diagonally cut into ½-inch slices

Directions: Pour 3 cups cold water into the bottom of a deep steamer pan. If you are using a shallow steamer, use only 2 cups. Thoroughly wash chicken breasts. Mix curry powder and 1 tsp of the dried dill and sprinkle over the chicken. Place chicken breasts in top of steamer pan, above water level. Layer the vegetables on top of the chicken. Sprinkle remaining tsp of dried dill over vegetables and cover pan with a tight-fitting lid. Bring water to a full boil and then reduce heat so that water continues to simmer and steam. Steam for 30 minutes, without removing the lid, until chicken is fully cooked.

ASIAN CABBAGE SALAD (BHD, FBD, HHD)

Serves 1

Ingredients:

- Small head Napa cabbage, thinly sliced
- 1 carrot
- 2 green onions
- 2 tbs shelled hemp seeds
- ¼ lb fresh snow peas
- ¼ cup sliced almonds
- 2 tbs low-fat Asian sesame dressing

Directions: Cut snow peas and green onion into small pieces and shred carrot. Mix all the ingredients together in large bowl and toss with dressing.

SHRIMP STUFFED PORTOBELLO CAPS (BHD, FBD, HHD)

Serves 4

Ingredients:

- 2 tsp extra-virgin olive oil
- 4 large Portobello mushroom caps (each about 5-inch diameter)
- 8 cups baby spinach leaves
- 1 medium red pepper
- 2 green onions
- 2 tbs rice flour
- ¼ tsp Old Bay Seasoning
- Salt to taste
- 8 "extra jumbo"–sized shrimp
- 1 fresh lemon
- Tabasco if desired

Directions: Preheat oven to 375°F. Prepare a shallow baking dish by spreading the olive oil over the bottom of the dish. Wash and remove gills from mushroom caps. Chop spinach, dice pepper and green onion. Mix the vegetables together. Divide equally and fill each mushroom cap with this mixture. In a separate bowl, mix rice flour, seasoning, and salt together. Peel and devein the shrimp. Dredge each shrimp in flour until coated and place on top of spinach mixture in each mushroom cap. Thinly slice lemon and place two or three slices on top of shrimp. Place the stuffed mushrooms in a baking dish and cover with aluminum foil. Bake for 35 to 40 minutes. Transfer to platter and sprinkle with Tabasco sauce if desired.

GRILLED PORTOBELLO AND EGGPLANT WRAP (BHD, FBD, HHD)

Serves 4

Ingredients:

- Nonstick olive oil spray
- 4 medium Portobello mushroom caps
- 2 large red bell peppers, quartered with seeds and stem removed
- 1 large tomato
- 1 medium-large eggplant
- 1 tbs crushed garlic
- 4 tbs olive oil mayonnaise
- 2 tbs lemon juice
- ½ tsp fresh horseradish
- 2 cups pumpkin seeds (shelled, unsalted)
- 4 large swiss chard or collard green leaves (large stem removed)
- Salt and pepper to taste

Directions: Preheat grill to medium-high. Remove the stems and gills from the mushroom caps with a large spoon. Slice the eggplant, mushrooms, and tomato into thick slices. Lightly spray all the vegetables with nonstick olive oil spray. Grill the vegetables until just tender and lightly browned on each side (between 2 and 4 minutes per side). Remove from grill and cut all vegetables into ½-inch cubes. In a large bowl, mix the mayonnaise, lemon juice, horseradish, and garlic until smooth. Toss the vegetables and pumpkin seeds with the mayonnaise mixture. Blanch the Swiss chard leaves in a skillet filled with ½ inch of boiling water for 2 minutes. This brings out the green color and makes the leaves pliable and easy to roll. Using 2 leaves for each wrap, place ½ to 1 cup of vegetable mixture in center of leaves and roll.

BARBECUE TUNA STEAKS (BHD, FBD, HHD)

Serves 4

Ingredients:

- 1 lb yellow fin tuna steaks cut into 4 even pieces
- 4 tbs olive oil mayonnaise
- 3 tbs fresh cilantro, chopped
- 1 tbs chili powder
- 2 cloves crushed garlic
- Juice from 1 lime

Directions: Heat grill or broiler. Blend mayonnaise, cilantro, lime juice, chili powder, and garlic. Let stand 20 minutes. Spread mayo mixture evenly on both sides of each tuna steak. Grill 4 to 6 minutes or until tuna begins to flake on each side.

BAKED SALMON ROLLS (BHD, FBD, HHD)

Serves 6

Ingredients:

4 to 6 cups fresh baby spinach

4 cloves garlic (thinly sliced)

½ cup slivered water chestnuts

1 cup thinly sliced mushrooms

6 salmon fillets (4 oz each)

Olive oil cooking spray

Fresh-ground pepper

Directions: Preheat oven to 400°F. Mix spinach, water chestnuts, garlic, and mushrooms together in bowl. Lightly coat baking dish or cookie sheet with olive oil spray. Place salmon on prepared dish. Divide spinach mixture evenly on each fillet and roll, securing the roll with a long toothpick or kitchen twine. Top each roll with freshly ground pepper as desired. Bake 8 to 10 minutes or until fish flakes easily when fork is inserted.

ANNIE'S VEGETARIAN WRAP-FOR-LIFE (BHD, FBD, HHD)

Serves 1

Ingredients:

1 large Swiss chard or collard green leaf

¼ cup red pepper, chopped

¼ cup zucchini, chopped or shredded

¼ cup chopped cilantro

¼ cup chopped tomatoes

¼ cup canned red kidney beans, drained

¼ cup canned garbanzo beans, drained

1 tbs chili powder

Directions: Blanch the leaf in a skillet filled with ½ inch of boiling water for 2 minutes. This brings out the green color and makes the leaf pliable and easy to roll. Meanwhile, mix all remaining ingredients together. Carefully slice the leaf in half along the stem, discarding the stem. Place half of the mixture on each half of the leaf and roll.

VEGAN CHILI (BHD, FBD, HHD)

Serves 6

Ingredients:

- 1 large white onion
- 1 green bell pepper
- 1 yellow bell pepper
- 1 red bell pepper
- 2 cups diced celery
- 1 cup fresh cilantro, chopped
- 6 Morningstar Farms® black bean burgers
- 1 (15-oz) can black beans, rinsed and drained
- 1 (15-oz) can great northern or cannellini beans, rinsed and drained
- 1 (15-oz) can dark red kidney beans, rinsed and drained
- 1 (28-oz) can diced tomatoes
- 2 cups vegetable broth
- ⅓ cup chili powder
- Red pepper flakes

Directions: Wash and dice onion, peppers, and celery. Chop cilantro and set aside. Put all the beans in a colander and thoroughly rinse and drain. Cut frozen black bean burgers into bite-size pieces and set aside. Pour just enough of the vegetable broth to cover the bottom of an 8- to 12-quart stock pot and heat over medium heat until barely bubbling. Add the onion and sauté just until it appears slightly opaque but still firm; approximately 3 minutes. All at once, add the peppers, celery, and cilantro and mix thoroughly. Cook over medium heat, stirring often, for about 5 minutes. Add the chili powder and remaining vegetable broth and stir. Add the beans, diced tomatoes, and black bean burger pieces and lightly stir the pot until all ingredients are mixed. Cook for an additional 10 minutes or until thoroughly heated. Add red pepper flakes to taste and serve.

ASIAN BEANS WITH HEMP SEEDS (BHD, FBD, HHD)

Serves 2

Ingredients:

- 1 lb fresh green beans, stems cut off and blanched
- 2 cloves minced garlic
- 1 shallot, diced
- 1 tbs sesame oil
- 1 tsp hot chili oil
- 1 tbs extra-virgin olive oil
- ½ cup shelled hemp seeds
- 3 tbs low-sodium soy sauce
- 1 tsp freshly grated ginger
- Juice from ½ fresh lemon
- Red pepper flakes, optional

Directions: Bring 3 quarts of water to a boil and immerse beans for 1 minute. Remove beans and plunge into ice water to stop the cooking process. Set aside. Heat large skillet over medium-low heat, add oils until just hot. Sauté the shallots, garlic, and ginger root until soft. Add beans and hemp seeds and stir until tender but still crunchy. Stir in soy sauce and lemon juice and cook for 1 more minute. Sprinkle with red pepper flakes, if desired.

LENTIL AND BEAN SALAD (BHD, FBD, HHD)

Serves 4

Ingredients:

- 1 (15-oz) can lentils
- 1 (15-oz) can cannellini beans
- 1 tbs extra-virgin olive oil
- 2 tbs diced red bell pepper
- 2 tbs diced green bell pepper
- 1 tbs diced red onion
- 1 tbs diced Italian parsley
- 1 tsp balsamic vinegar
- 2 cups fresh greens

Directions: Rinse and drain lentils and beans and set aside. In a large skillet, add olive oil, peppers, and onions and sauté over medium heat until just tender (about 2 minutes). All at once, add the beans and lentils and stir until sufficiently heated. Remove from heat and stir in parsley and vinegar. Serve over greens for a filling and healthy salad.

DIJON SALMON (BHD, FBD, HHD)

Serves 6

Ingredients:

Nonstick cooking spray

6 salmon fillets (4 oz each)

1 medium red onion, sliced

Fresh parsley sprigs

Marinade:

¾ cup Dijon mustard

2 tsp red pepper flakes

1 tbs red wine vinegar

1 tbs extra-virgin olive oil

Directions: To prepare the marinade, mix mustard, red pepper, vinegar, and olive oil in a large bowl. Add salmon fillets and marinate for 30 minutes, turning once. Heat grill or broiler. Prepare grill skillet or flat grid by spraying lightly with nonstick cooking spray. Place fillets on grid and brush with marinade. Broil or grill 5 to 7 minutes. Turn fillets and cook for an additional 5 to 7 minutes or until salmon flakes easily with fork.

HEALTHY GREENS AND BEANS (BHD, FBD, HHD)

Serves 4

Ingredients:

1 can (15 oz) cannellini beans

2 cups fresh collard greens, chopped

2 cups fresh kale, chopped

2 red bell peppers, coarsely chopped

3 cups diced fresh tomatoes

1 cup diced onion

2 cloves garlic, crushed

1 cup fat-free, low-sodium vegetable broth

Balsamic vinegar to taste

Directions: Rinse and drain cannellini beans and set aside. In a large pot, bring 6 cups water to a full boil. Add the greens to the water and boil for 3 minutes. Drain immediately and rinse under cold water. In a large skillet over medium heat, combine broth, onion, tomatoes, peppers, and garlic. Simmer 8 to 10 minutes or until onions are opaque. Add the cooked greens and beans and simmer for another 4 minutes. Season with a sprinkle of balsamic vinegar.

VEGETARIAN STUFFED PEPPERS (BHD, FBD, HHD)

Serves 4

Ingredients:

- 4 large red or yellow bell peppers
- Olive oil cooking spray
- 1½ cups fat-free, low-sodium vegetable broth
- 4 cups (loosely packed) chopped kale
- 4 cups (loosely packed) chopped collard greens
- 1 small minced onion
- ¼ cup chopped red pimento
- 3 cloves minced garlic
- ½ cup chopped walnuts
- ¼ cup chia seeds
- ½ lemon
- 1½ cups cooked wild rice
- Coarse ground pepper

Directions: Heat oven to 400°F. Cut bell peppers in half lengthwise and remove seeds. Lightly spray bottom of deep baking dish with cooking spray. Place peppers open side down in dish and bake for 12 minutes or until just tender. Remove and allow to cool. In a large pot bring 1 cup of water and the vegetable broth to a boil. Add kale and collard greens and cover with tight-fitting lid. Reduce heat to medium and cook greens for 10 to 12 minutes. Drain and set aside. Lightly spray large skillet with cooking spray and heat over medium heat. Sauté onion, garlic, and pimento until just tender. Add nuts and squeeze a small amount of lemon juice over contents of skillet. Add cooked greens and sauté until heated. Remove from heat; stir in rice and chia seeds. Fill pepper halves with greens and rice mixture. Season with ground pepper if desired. Place stuffed peppers in baking dish and cover with lid or aluminum foil. Return to oven and bake for approximately 20 to 25 minutes or until thoroughly heated.

HERB-RUBBED PORK TENDERLOIN (HHD, FBD)

Substitute seitan loaf for HHD.

Serves 4

Ingredients:

1 tsp dried thyme

1 tsp dried rosemary

½ tsp garlic powder

1 slice Ezekiel bread

2 egg whites, lightly beaten

1 (1-lb) pork tenderloin, trimmed

¼ tsp salt

¼ tsp freshly ground black pepper

Cooking spray

Directions: Preheat oven to 400°F. Place thyme, rosemary, garlic powder, and Ezekiel bread in a food processor; pulse until fine. Measure out ⅓ cup of breadcrumbs and place in a shallow dish. Place egg whites in a second shallow dish. Sprinkle pork with salt and pepper. Dip pork in egg whites; dredge in breadcrumbs. Place pork on a broiler pan coated with cooking spray. Bake for 30 minutes or until a thermometer registers 155°. Let stand 5 minutes. Cut into ¼-inch-thick slices.

HIGH-PROTEIN TURKEY MEATBALLS (HHD, FBD)

Serves 4

Ingredients:

1¼ lbs turkey breast, ground

1 red pepper, diced

1 onion, diced

1 cup mushrooms, chopped

3 egg whites

¼ tsp onion powder

¼ tsp garlic powder

Directions: Preheat oven to 375°F. Mix all ingredients together. Form into meatballs (about 2 inches in diameter). Bake on cookie sheet for 40 minutes.

SCALLOP AND WHITE BEAN GUMBO (HHD, FBD)

Omit scallops and double the beans for HHD. Another great make-ahead recipe that can last you all week.

Serves 7

Ingredients:

- ½ cup olive oil
- ⅓ cup whole wheat flour
- 1 onion, chopped
- 1 green bell pepper, chopped
- 2 celery stalks, chopped
- 2 tbs minced garlic
- 1 tsp salt
- ¼ tsp black pepper
- 2½ cups low-fat chicken stock, unsalted
- 2 cups tomatoes, chopped
- 1 tbs fresh thyme
- 1 tbs fresh oregano
- 1 bay leaf
- 1 jalapeno pepper (optional), seeds removed and thinly sliced
- 1 (15-oz) can cannellini beans, rinsed and drained
- 1 lb scallops

Directions: Put oil in a large pot over medium-low heat. Add flour and cook, stirring almost constantly, about 15 to 20 minutes; as it cooks, adjust heat to keep mixture from burning. Add onion, bell pepper, celery, and garlic and raise heat to medium. Sprinkle with salt and pepper and cook, stirring frequently, until vegetables have softened. Stir in the stock, tomatoes, thyme, oregano, bay leaf, and jalapeno. Cover, bring to a boil, then reduce heat so soup bubbles steadily. Cook for about 20 minutes. Add beans and scallops and cook until scallops are opaque and firm, about 2 minutes. Remove bay leaf before serving.

SCALLOP AND AVOCADO RICE BOWL (HHD, FBD)

Replace scallops with tofu for HHD.

Serves 4

Ingredients:

- 16 medium scallops, cleaned and thawed if frozen
- 1 tsp sesame oil
- Pinch cayenne pepper
- 1 tbs light soy sauce
- 1 tbs rice wine vinegar
- 1 cup shelled edamame, steamed
- 2 tsp toasted shelled hemp seeds
- 1¼ cups brown rice, cooked according to package directions
- 1 ripe avocado, sliced

Directions: Preheat the broiler. In a medium ovenproof pan, toss the scallops with 1 tsp of sesame oil and cayenne. Lay the scallops flat on a broiler pan and cook for 2 minutes per side. Transfer to a plate. In a small bowl, combine the soy sauce and rice wine vinegar. Add the edamame and hemp seeds to the rice. Divide the avocado into 4 servings. Serve the rice in bowls topped with the scallops and avocado. Drizzle the soy-vinegar mixture before serving.

PORK CHOPS WITH CHERRIES AND ALMONDS (HHD, FBD)

Serves 4

Ingredients:

- 2 tbs olive oil
- 4 (5-oz) bone-in center-cut pork chops
- 1 tsp salt
- Cooking spray
- 1 cup coarsely chopped pitted cherries
- ½ cup sliced green onions
- ⅓ cup almonds, chopped
- 2 tbs fresh lemon juice

Directions: Preheat grill or broiler. Lightly brush olive oil evenly over both sides of pork. Place pork on a grill rack coated with cooking spray and grill 4 minutes on each side or until desired degree of doneness is reached. Let pork stand for 5 minutes. Meanwhile, in a large bowl, combine remaining ingredients, adding a drizzle of olive oil to hold together. Serve on top of pork.

Shake Variations

These shakes are delicious and add variety without adding lots of calories. Try them all and use them as snacks or breakfast options, along with the plain varieties listed in the meal plans. The directions are always the same: Combine ingredients in a blender filled with ice. You can add or remove ice to achieve your desired thickness. Shakes can use a variety of protein sources, such as whey, casein, egg, soy, and milk: All are available at health food stores or on the Internet. My favorites are whey and casein. Casein is absorbed slowly so it is really great at preventing "nighttime munchies." Whey is absorbed much faster and I use it first thing in the morning, right after I work out with weights.

CHOCOLATE PEANUT BUTTER SHAKE

Chocolate protein shake powder (prepare as directed)
1 tbs all-natural peanut butter

ANY BERRY SHAKE

Protein shake powder (plain; prepare as directed)
1 cup mixed berries (fresh or frozen—no sugar added)

BLUEBERRY VANILLA SHAKE

Vanilla protein shake powder (prepare as directed)
½ cup fresh or frozen blueberries (no sugar added)

CHOCOLATE ALMOND PROTEIN SHAKE

Chocolate protein shake powder (prepare as directed)
¼ cup fresh almonds

MY FAVORITE BREAKFAST SHAKE

4 ice cubes

½ cup of low-fat half-&-half

⅔ cup cold coffee

1½ scoops of chocolate whey protein powder

VANILLA WALNUT CITRUS SHAKE

1 scoop vanilla protein powder

1 orange, peeled and sectioned

¼ orange peel

2 tbs walnuts

1 cup low-fat cottage cheese (use soy yogurt for FBD or HHD)

1½ cups water

CHOCOLATE CHERRY SHAKE

1½ cups cherries, pitted (frozen or fresh)

2 tbs walnuts, chopped

2 scoops chocolate protein powder

1 tbs unsweetened cocoa powder

1½ cups water

CARROT GINGER SHAKE

1 cup soy or low-fat milk

1 scoop protein powder

2 tbs peanut butter

1 tbs hemp seeds

1 tbs chia seeds

1 tsp cinnamon

¼ tsp ground ginger

1 large carrot, shredded

GINGER PEAR SHAKE

1 scoop protein powder

1 cup water

½ tbs hemp seeds

2 tbs chopped fresh ginger

¼ cup soy or low-fat milk

1 pear, peeled and sliced

1 cup spinach

FRUIT AND TEA SHAKE

2 cups green rooibos tea, steeped and chilled (substitute plain green tea or your favorite herbal choice)

1 scoop protein powder

1 cup frozen blueberries

2 tbs hemp seeds

MYSTICAL MINT WHEY SHAKE

1 cup cold water

1 tbs almonds, raw, slivered

1 scoop whey protein chocolate powder

1 tsp peppermint extract

PART THREE

FEELING YOUNGER EVERY YEAR

CHAPTER 12

Hormones and Nutraceuticals: A Potential Factor for Weight Loss

The second prong of the Life Plan Diet is to support your efforts with the best that modern medicine has to offer. That means making sure that your hormone levels fall within a healthy range and choosing nutraceuticals—vitamin and mineral supplements—that actually do what they claim and really improve health and your chances of trimming down your belly fat.

The Why and How of Hormone Therapies

The loss of testosterone and other hormones that the male human body naturally produces is referred to as *andropause*. Some say it is the male equivalent to menopause, and I both agree and disagree. It's true that it refers to a hormonal loss, which is what defines menopause. But women experience a much more abrupt and obvious decline in hormonal production, and therefore have significant symptoms as a result. For men, this hormonal decrease is slow and insidious, taking place over many years, and is so subtle that you won't notice that it's happening until you are several years into it.

As a result, men are at a real disadvantage as they begin to struggle with serious symptoms: Because the hormonal drop is slow and steady, the signs and symptoms of andropause are sometimes imperceptible until bigger health problems emerge. Beyond the declining sexual function, and the health issues we reviewed in Chapter 1, the two most prominent symptoms of andropause are higher body fat (especially belly fat) and loss of energy. This means that if you are over the age of 40 and are following the Life Plan Diet religiously, your best efforts may be compromised by andropause.

Five years after winning the 1998 Body-for-LIFE contest, I noticed that I was gaining body fat and losing strength, despite eating clean and exercising vigorously. Diagnostic bloodwork revealed my testosterone levels were at the bottom of the reference range. So my physician started me on testosterone therapy, and I've never looked back. Within two months I began feeling a remarkable change: more strength, better muscle mass, improved sexual function, higher energy levels, reduced cholesterol, good blood sugar control, clearer thinking, and a renewed zest for life. I know that there's no way I could accomplish all that I do every day at 75 if I wasn't combining diet and exercise with correcting my hormone deficiencies.

But that's me. You have to examine your own health issues and goals. I'm here to help you on that journey with the only thing I can give you: good advice, better science, and the absolute truth about what hormone therapies can do for your health and your current level of fatness.

First of all, it's a common misconception that using growth hormone and testosterone replacement therapies is the same as steroid abuse by athletes. The confusion comes from a simple twist to the equation: When used properly by men who have a known clinical deficiency, these therapies are safe, useful, and an effective way to reduce and reverse disease and improve quality of life. However, when athletes in their twenties and thirties are taking the same medications without having a deficiency, and undoubtedly taking way too much, and they are not being carefully monitored by a physician, these same medicines can be dangerous to their health while enabling them to cheat at their sport.

Professional, elite athletes may believe that using testosterone and growth hormone therapies will increase strength and improve their performance. Because their use is not well monitored, these athletes can take excessive doses of testosterone and growth hormone, which increase their blood levels 10 to 20 times above the upper limits of the normal reference range. It is also unclear whether such abuse actually improves athletic prowess. We do know that it will allow athletes to recover from injury faster, but only if there has been a clearly defined deficiency.

The proper and approved use of testosterone and growth hormone therapies for the treatment of hormone deficiencies has been supported by countless evidence-based scientific studies published over the past 10 years in well-respected, peer-reviewed medical journals. I've reviewed the science countless times in my other books, *The Life Plan* and *Mastering the Life Plan*, but I've included the research references in this book just so that you can show your own doctor that this is not "quackery." In fact, it is widely accepted that hormone deficiencies are a major factor in accelerating the aging process and increasing risks for all of the age-related diseases that are killing most Americans prematurely. These treatments are completely legal for those who have been diagnosed as deficient, and can be prescribed by a doctor after appropriate clinical testing proves a deficiency. These therapies require constant medical supervision, and when they are monitored carefully and used religiously there are minimal side effects, if any.

A second myth surrounding these therapies is that they are responsible for building muscle and getting rid of body fat. This is not exactly the case. Hormone replacement therapy has helped me create an optimal environment within my body—a healthy blend of hormones that are at healthy levels that correct my own deficiencies—which has enabled me to maximize my training. If I didn't train and eat like I do, I wouldn't look like I do . . . I'd just be a fatter version of my "before" picture with better hormone levels. Hormone therapies allow deficient men to increase their metabolism and maintain weight loss, but the reason men like me look the way they do is that they spend time at the gym each day working out, and they eat "clean."

It is very likely that the same professional athletes who are abusing hormonal therapies are also working out at elite levels every day. These guys train so intensely that to some extent it's questionable whether their athletic performance really benefits from growth hormone or testosterone replacement therapy. I do believe that these therapies make them feel psychologically better and probably allow them to train harder and have fewer injuries. But whether it makes them better athletes is unclear.

This controversy isn't going away anytime soon. In 2014, the National Football League is hoping to begin a study of players and their possible use of hGH, and it may become an even murkier issue. It's quite likely that some football players may be appropriately using these therapies for real medical reasons and with complete medical supervision. It's also likely that many players may be doping to enhance their performance. Either way, we need to both address and understand these different uses so that we can legitimize the medical use of these therapies and punish the young players who may be abusing them.

Men Need Testosterone

Testosterone replacement therapy is frequently prescribed by doctors all over the world to address declining hormone levels in men. Decreased libido and erectile quality are the most frequent findings associated with falling testosterone levels, yet they are actually some of the latest symptoms, with other findings present much sooner, such as weight gain.

Studies have been done looking at the relationship between testosterone replacement and a return to a more favorable body composition. The consensus in the medical literature is that testosterone supplementation is accompanied by gains in lean mass across all age groups. It is associated with reduced body fat, with some preferential fat loss seen in the abdomen.

If you won't consider testing to improve your sex life or your waistline, think of your overall health. A man with low testosterone could face greater risk for heart disease, Alzheimer's, prostate cancer, and sarcopenia (loss of muscle mass or frailty associated with aging). Men with low testosterone have a 33 percent greater death risk over their next 18 years of life compared with men having higher testosterone.

The heart—and not the testicles—is the organ with the highest concentration of testosterone receptors. Testosterone is associated with several positive effects on cardiac health. It has been linked with reducing coronary artery disease (CAD) and hypertension risk as well as with improving cardiac function in patients with pre-existing heart disease. In large population studies it has been found that low testosterone levels are associated with increased risk of atherosclerotic cardiac disease. Older men treated with testosterone can show decreases in total cholesterol and LDL. Low testosterone levels also are correlated with a greater degree of atherosclerotic blockage when coronary artery disease is present.

The brain is second only to the heart in terms of abundance of testosterone receptors. Testosterone is associated with maintaining cognitive function, lowered dementia risk, and decreasing symptoms of depression, anxiety, and panic disorders. Maintaining testosterone levels carries a significant cognitive benefit.

Testosterone is also the key to fighting inflammation. Recent research from Friedrich Schiller University in Germany revealed an intriguing fact: Men and women do not respond to inflammatory stimuli in the same manner. It turns out that the enzyme phospholipase D—an inflammatory stimulant and regulator of critical aspects of cell physiology—is not as active in male cells as it is in female cells. Based on that, the study suggests that testosterone is pivotal to maintaining a proper immune response and protecting the body from inflammation. This is important because inflammation is the underlying cause of most chronic diseases related to aging. Finally, diminished hormones, particularly testosterone, put men at risk for debilitating conditions, such as hip fractures. In addition to correlating testosterone with declining bone density, it is also linked intimately with muscle loss.

If bad press is the only thing standing in the way of your achieving better health through testosterone therapy, let me be very clear: *There is no link between elevated testosterone levels and prostate cancer*. While testosterone is associated with prostate cancer risk, it is in the exact opposite relationship. Historically, doctors feared that raising testosterone levels might cause prostate cancer to grow. This fear stems from a 1941 journal article reporting that testosterone injections caused an enhanced rate of prostate growth, and castration caused prostate regression. Unfortunately, this study was conducted on only one patient. Further research, however, has failed to support this review. A large longitudinal study found no relationship between testosterone concentrations and the risk for prostate cancer, except to discover that one risk factor of prostate cancer was low testosterone levels, not high.

Why this myth keeps being circulated is beyond my comprehension, because the truth is, testosterone therapies are completely safe and effective. Some doctors continue to speak out against these therapies, saying that reversing hormone deficiencies is unsafe and, more to the point, "unnatural." I think it's perfectly natural to want to maintain a younger, healthier, more vibrant body and lifestyle at any age. I have a choice about how I'm going to manage my health, and so do you. You can choose to grow old and weak and fat, or you can choose to do something about it.

In terms of safety, the pharmaceutical industry has realized that testosterone therapy is big business, and has responded to increased demand by developing new methods for administering natural testosterone. Side effects are rare and typically occur during the first few months, but they usually resolve themselves. These can include skin reactions such as acne, oily skin, erythema, breast tenderness, erythrocytosis (increased production of red blood cells), COPD (chronic obstructive lung disease), sleep apnea, and lower-extremity edema (swelling).

You need to work with your current physician to come up with a program that optimizes your hormone levels. The first step is to obtain the proper testing. The first important blood test is called *total serum testosterone*, which is performed first thing in the morning. Some specialists, including myself, believe that you also need a *free or unbound testosterone level* check.

A skilled, experienced medical doctor who monitors blood testosterone levels and performs a digital rectal exam of your prostate along with PSA tests to screen for prostate cancer must administer your therapy. At my office, every man undergoes a highly comprehensive evaluation to first determine if a clinical hormone deficiency exists. Any man needing a correction of hormone deficiencies has bloodwork done at six weeks, and again every three to four months after that to ensure levels stay in the healthy range.

Because every man's hormone levels are unique, it's impossible to know exactly how high your levels were before they declined. What's more, not every man is a good candidate for testosterone therapy. Discuss your current health status with your doctor, especially if you have a history of obstructive sleep apnea or heart failure. If you do, you need to see an appropriate specialist before starting therapy. Most men require some fine-tuning of their treatment until the best results are achieved. You should notice that your symptoms begin to improve in three to six weeks after you start treatment.

There are many different ways to administer testosterone. These are the most popular:

Transdermal: Gels, creams, or patches. I'm not a fan of this approach. Its absorption can be affected by weather conditions and it can be transferred to your partner, or even your kids. Plus, you need to apply it daily.

Pellets: Surgically implanted into your muscles. This testosterone-delivery method slowly leaks into your system as it dissolves over a period of weeks. Problems arise if levels become too high; you'll need to have a pellet taken out. Low levels mean another pellet needs to be inserted.

Injections in the upper outer buttocks or upper lateral thigh: This is my preferred method, because it allows you to see your doctor regularly so that he or she can stay on top of your levels and keep them at a healthy, steady state.

Under the tongue (twice daily): This method of testosterone administration has not been studied well and carries with it a potential risk of serious side effects.

Create More T on Your Own

You can increase your own testosterone production naturally, and if you've already been following the Life Plan Diet, you may be well on your way. Studies clearly show that losing excess body fat, especially around and in your belly, is enormously beneficial, since belly fat produces estrogen, which competes with testosterone receptors throughout your body. Without available receptors, it doesn't matter how much testosterone you produce.

We also know that the way you take off excess body fat matters when it comes to maintaining testosterone levels. Extremely low-fat diets result in low testosterone levels, and diets like mine that are higher in protein, lower in carbohydrates, and moderate in fats result in the greatest sustained high levels of testosterone. This is why men must eat plenty of lean protein: It stimulates the hormone glucagon and other muscle-building responses important for increased testosterone release. Low-glycemic carbs found in fruits and vegetables lower insulin and cortisol levels, which not only make you feel bloated but interfere with testosterone production. The essential fatty acids (omega-3s) found in fish that we discussed early are also essential for the body to produce testosterone. And because the Life Plan Diet is not extremely caloric deficient, it won't trick your body into thinking that it's starving, which would send testosterone levels plummeting.

Both a lack of and an excess in physical activity will decrease your testosterone levels. Testosterone actually decreases during extended periods of endurance training. After 60 minutes of exercise, cortisol levels begin to rise and testosterone levels decrease as a result of overtraining. This decrease can last up to six days. However, testosterone levels can increase when you are following an exercise program that is short and very intense. Strength-training large muscle groups does the best job of raising testosterone. For a complete strength-training workout that's optimized for increasing muscle and decreasing belly fat, you can follow the plans I've outlined in my previous books.

Other lifestyle changes can help increase your testosterone levels. Make sure you get a full eight hours of sleep as often as possible to maximize your testosterone production. Hormone production is greatest when your body is at rest, which is another reason it's important to get plenty of good sleep. Avoiding cigarettes, minimizing the use of alcohol, and controlling the stress in your life are also beneficial to testosterone production.

The Role of Growth Hormone

I also have strong feelings about human growth hormone therapies, because I have witnessed remarkable reversals in aging and disease by using it myself. At the same time, the medical community and the media continue to get this one all wrong. I also want to make it very clear that like any type of medicine, it should not be abused, and it should be used only when it is determined to be absolutely necessary—that is, to deal with a documented deficiency. Growth hormone therapies are critical for adults with this relatively rare medical condition to reverse many of the major effects of aging, including muscle loss, weakness, skin tone and texture, excess body fat deposits, energy depletion, and declining immune function. Cardiovascular disease, stroke, and obesity are all related to a growth hormone deficiency.

Human growth hormone is naturally produced by the pituitary gland in the brain and is critical for repair throughout your body. Preventive medicine specialists like me have embraced human growth hormone (hGH) as a treatment option for adults with clinically proven deficiencies. It was first developed to aid in growth for children of small stature, and it is still prescribed for this purpose by endocrinologists today. Before 1986, human growth hormone was harvested from cadavers and carried a risk of transmission of disease to its recipients. Since then, growth hormone has been commercially produced in laboratories by major pharmaceutical firms and issues concerning disease transmission are no longer applicable: hGH is safe, available, and easy to administer.

As we age, our growth hormone production decreases. Adult hGH levels decline by half from ages 20 to 60, and the loss accelerates thereafter. The typical decline begins at age 40, and one of the telltale symptoms is abdominal obesity. Other symptoms include:

- Decreased libido

- Decreased muscular strength

- Depression

- Diabetes

- Dyslipidemia (abnormal cholesterol panel)

- Endothelial dysfunction

- Fatigue

- Hypertension

- Hypothyroidism

- Memory loss

- Metabolic syndrome

- Osteoporosis

- Poor cognitive stability

- Reduced exercise capacity

- Sarcopenia

- Sleep apnea

- Sleep disturbance

What hGH Therapy Looks Like

Human growth hormone is expensive and in most cases is not covered by health insurance policies, but if you have a clinical deficiency and you cannot lose body fat, no matter how hard you try, you might want to explore this therapy. Numerous studies of growth hormone replacement therapy have found that this form of treatment decreases fat mass and increases lean body mass in deficient individuals.

Current clinical guidelines from the Endocrine Society state that there is no evidence that the incidence of tumors is increased by growth hormone therapy, even though some of the media have clung to this as a potential risk factor. In 2001, the Growth Hormone

Research Society extensively reviewed the question of whether growth hormone therapy is associated with tumor growth. Their final statement was clear: For patients receiving growth hormone therapy, "No additional monitoring for other malignant tumors (such as tumors of the prostate, breast, or colon) is currently suggested beyond the accepted standard of care for the patient's age and sex."

This does not mean that every man gets the green light when it comes to this therapy. You must test positively for a clinical deficiency in order to get a prescription for this medication. Doctors like me who administer growth hormone must adhere to state and federal guidelines. The gold standard for diagnosing a growth hormone deficiency has been the *insulin tolerance test (ITT):* It is the same stimulation test used by many endocrinologists. Another stimulation test is the *glucagon stimulation test,* which is considered much safer than the ITT. Many investigators and clinicians reject the ITT and other stimulation tests for diagnosing adult growth hormone deficiency and rely on a blood test called IGF-1 as a more reliable diagnostic and therapeutic marker of growth hormone deficiency.

In spite of all this controversy, the FDA and hGH manufacturers have maintained their positions that stimulation testing is necessary and required for an accurate diagnosis. In my practice, I use glucagon pituitary stimulation testing as a prerequisite for diagnosing growth hormone deficiency. Once therapy begins, all of my patients receiving hGH must be followed closely with repeat blood draws every four to five months to ensure that their levels are in the correct range and markers of disease are improving.

If you follow the Life Plan Diet for eight weeks and your growth hormone levels remain low and the signs and symptoms have not improved, I would suggest that you undergo a stimulation test to confirm your suspicion of growth hormone deficiency.

Improve Your Production of Growth Hormone

Healthy lifestyle choices enable you to increase your own production of human growth hormone. hGH is measured as IGF-1 (Insulin-like Growth Factor 1). As the name implies, "Insulin-like Growth Factor 1" is structurally related to insulin. These two hormones share the same receptor sites on cells, creating a competition in which only one hormone will be predominantly effective. A nutrition program that focuses on keeping insulin levels as low as possible will enable you to increase your own natural production of IGF-1.

Because you need to optimize growth hormone levels and IGF-1 levels, my diet is designed to keep blood sugars low, allowing you to effectively manage your insulin, which will help you achieve healthy levels of growth hormone and IGF-1 on your own. That's why I know that following a comprehensive diet program like this one is the first step to creating more growth hormone as well as testosterone. I'm very pleased when my patients follow my protocol and come back to my office after just eight weeks with significant increases in their growth hormone levels. Once the body learns to do this, it will continue increased production as you continue the program.

Your bad eating habits may have been one of the reasons your body is not producing the proper levels of growth hormone. A high-saturated-fat, high-glycemic diet reduces growth hormone secretion by 30 percent. However, following a low-glycemic diet high in lean proteins and healthy fats can increase your levels. Amino acids such as arginine, found in all protein sources, stimulate growth hormone secretion. Positive correlations have also been shown between growth hormone production and the intake of micronutrients such as calcium, iron, potassium, magnesium, niacin, phosphorus, riboflavin, thiamine, and zinc found in vegetables, fruits, and nutraceuticals. While the Life Plan Diet was initially developed for heart health, the growth hormone benefits are equally important.

We produce growth hormone all day long, but mostly during deep sleep. Men who don't sleep well or don't sleep enough will invariably have low levels of growth hormone, and many will be growth hormone deficient.

Exercise can play a significant role in growth hormone secretion. About 10 to 20 minutes of aerobic exercise causes a rise in serum levels that peak at the end of that period and are sustained for up to two hours. This means that if you have been walking as directed in the program, you are already improving your growth hormone levels. If you take your exercise to the next step and start incorporating resistance training, you'll increase your levels even more.

Other Hormones to Consider

Your physician will help you come up with a program that optimizes all of your hormone levels: You can't just pick and choose which ones you want to work on. There is a wide range of hormones that you can consider replacing, depending on your current health status and deficiencies you may have. However, not all hormone therapies are the same. Synthetic hormones such as methyltestosterone carry a black box warning connecting it to liver cancer. It has also been shown that growth hormones harvested from cadavers cause cancer.

I prescribe only pharmaceutically approved hormones, which are plant-based, natural, and safe. These hormones produce the same physiological responses as the body's own natural hormones. I commonly prescribe for men the following:

DHEA (dehydroepiandrosterone): Produced in the adrenal cortex of the adrenal gland as well as the testicles. It is then converted to estrogen and testosterone. Re-establishing DHEA balance to more youthful levels can enhance sexual desire, performance, and overall mood. It is also used for increasing production of testosterone and growth hormone, as well as combatting chronic fatigue syndrome, depression, memory loss, and osteoporosis. DHEA is so mild that it can be purchased over the counter as a supplement, but I recommend pharmaceutical-grade DHEA to make sure you are really getting what you are paying for. I have tested many of my patients taking inferior DHEA products and found, not surprisingly, low blood levels.

Thyroid (T3 and/or T4): Some men experiencing sexual dysfunction may actually have underlying thyroid disease. When we correct these deficiencies, they not only feel better, they also perform better in bed. These hormones can also help relieve depression, brain fog, fatigue, and other age-related symptoms. Thyroid hormone therapies can be obtained only with a doctor's prescription.

Melatonin: Supplementing with melatonin helps regulate sleep patterns, but it also has antioxidant properties for overall health and protection from cancer. Melatonin can help you relax, so it may also improve sexual performance. This can be purchased over the counter as a supplement. It has a short half-life of only two or three hours, so I recommend sustained-release formulations.

Supplements Beyond Hormone Therapies

Unlike hormone therapies, which are controlled substances that require a prescription, the supplement or nutraceutical industry is like the Wild West of medicine. Almost anything goes, especially if there is marketing money behind it. The variability among producers, brand names, and even types of supplements can make even the most levelheaded man's brain burst. So let me give you a quick run-through of all your options, and then I'll focus on the few that I find to be the most effective.

Types of Supplementation

There are two major groups of supplements. The first I'll refer to as *essential nutrients*, which are replacements for crucial vitamins and minerals that your body must have in order to function properly. These include vitamins and minerals, essential fatty acids, and probiotics.

Vitamins are organic compounds, meaning that they come from living things, such as plants or animals. They are necessary for proper bodily functioning, and we need only very small amounts of them. However, our bodies cannot manufacture sufficient quantities of them on our own. Instead, we have to get them from the foods we eat. In order to ensure that people get the right amounts of certain vitamins, U.S. government regulations require that some processed foods be fortified with vitamins. These include milk and dairy products, breakfast cereals, and grains.

Minerals are inorganic elements that come from the soil and water and are then absorbed by plants or animals that we eat. Our bodies need large amounts of some minerals, such as calcium, and very small amounts of other minerals, such as selenium and chromium, to stay healthy.

Essential fatty acids (EFAs) are compounds that are necessary for optimal health, yet we cannot make them in our bodies and must, therefore, consume them from high-fat foods. There are two basic types: omega-6 fatty acids, found in cooking oils, and omega-3 fatty acids, found in fatty fish and some plants. Omega-3 fatty acids have anti-inflammatory effects and are helpful for combatting inflammatory diseases such as rheumatoid arthritis. They are also considered protective against heart disease. Americans consume roughly 10 times more omega-6 fatty acids than omega-3 fatty acids. These large amounts of omega-6 fatty acids produce an unhealthy imbalance in the omega-3-to-omega-6 fatty acid ratio, which is thought to be a contributing factor for heart and blood vessel disease. To strike a better balance, we need to increase our consumption of omega-3 fatty acids, and one way to do this is through dietary supplements of high-quality fish oil capsules. You will definitely have to consider taking these when you are following the Heart Health Diet, because the foods and cooking methods on the plan have very little omega-3 fat.

Finally, probiotics are living microorganisms similar to what is normally found in the human gut. They are also referred to as "friendly bacteria" or "good bacteria." Probiotics may help with a number of health issues, including GI distress, symptoms of lactose intolerance, inflammation, cancer prevention, and enhanced micronutrient absorption.

Of these four categories, only some vitamins and probiotics are found in the body, although as we get older, we tend to produce lower quantities. Yet all four types of essential nutrients are necessary to good health. Supplementing these nutrients have been studied in both short-term and longitudinal research and has demonstrated overwhelming efficacy for a variety of health concerns. For example, a vitamin D deficiency is linked to all kinds of accelerated aging; fish oil supplementation reduces your risk for vascular diseases that lead to heart attacks and strokes; and many vitamins work together to improve immune function and protect the body against many cancers.

Several years ago scientists thought that supplementing with vitamins and minerals was necessary only to prevent diseases such as scurvy, pellagra, and rickets—diseases we rarely hear about today. Now nutritional experts fully understand that these same micronutrients play key roles in the prevention of heart disease, cancer, arthritis, and cataracts, along with the signs and symptoms of aging, including loss of muscle mass, strength, and bone mass. Supplementing your diet guarantees that you have every advantage in order to optimize health, fight disease, improve libido, sharpen the mind, stabilize blood sugar/insulin, and maintain energy levels so that you can work out vigorously and still have plenty of stamina for the rest of the day.

Regardless of how healthily we eat, supplementing with quality nutraceuticals is critical for everybody, especially men. Soils have long been depleted of vitamins and minerals from years of overfarming, chemical toxins, and acid rain. And, even if you ate only organic foods that are thought to be higher in vitamins and minerals, most men do not consume sufficient amounts of the many nutrients we need from the foods we eat, even if we follow a careful diet.

Oxidative stress is another very important reason that active men need to make sure that they are getting the right amount of micronutrients. "Oxidation" is the term used for the process of removing electrons from an atom or molecule. The result of this change can be destructive: For example, rust occurs on iron as it is exposed to oxygen. The same process can occur throughout the body. As we create energy by burning digested food with the oxygen we breathe, this process enables us to create a lean, muscular, healthy body.

However, excess oxygen can produce dangerous by-products, which include free radicals. Free radicals are the electrically unstable oxygen molecules that must scavenge electrons from whatever sources they can to become stable molecules. The sources of these scavenged electrons can include DNA, cell membranes, important enzymes, and vital structural or functional proteins. When these important cell parts and substances lose their electrons to free radicals, their function is altered, and the results can be catastrophic—cancer, heart disease, dementia, arthritis, muscle damage, increased susceptibility to infection, and accelerated aging.

The good news is that the fix is relatively easy. Antioxidants found in colorful fruits and vegetables can help protect us from these free radicals. Supplementation with relatively high doses of the known antioxidants, which includes vitamins C, E, and A, the mineral selenium, and phytochemicals, is probably the most reasonable way to address this issue.

However, when it comes to taking supplemental vitamins, more is not always better. Some vitamins are actually dangerous if consumed in high dosages. For example, too much vitamin A can lead to toxicity and bone loss. Some are more effective when they are kept refrigerated, including probiotics such as acidophilus. And some may interact with medications that you are currently taking, such as blood thinners. Always work with your doctor to determine the levels that you require. Start the discussion by mentioning the range I suggest below, and tailor it to your current weight and health status. Make sure your doctor knows all of your medications and that you are planning on following an intense exercise and nutrition program.

Remember, vitamins and minerals cannot cure a disease state, so they are not a substitute for prescription medications that you may be taking. Rather, they bolster your body's overall function so that over time, you may be able to lower the dosage of or eliminate some of your prescription drugs. For example, folate, better known as folic acid, is one of the B vitamins that is necessary for the healthy division of cells and the prevention of colon cancer. It can also play a key role in the growth of new muscle tissue that is essential to increasing muscle mass and strength. It also helps prevent heart and blood vessel disease by keeping homocystine levels low. A large government study in 2002 found that people who consumed the most folate had the fewest strokes and the least heart disease. This doesn't mean, however, that these people were able to stop taking their medication.

The second type of supplement group is now commonly referred to as *nutraceuticals*. This term was coined to refer to foods, or parts of food, including dietary supplements, that provide medical or health benefits, including the prevention and treatment of disease, in addition to their basic nutritional value. This category covers a wide swath, from energy bars and drinks to nutritional supplements in the forms of botanicals, teas, spices, and herbs, as well as compounds and formulations of dietary supplements. Though there have been many studies that can support the effectiveness of nutraceuticals, there have been an equal number that show these to be less than effective. Because of this, I'm cautious about many of these types of supplements. The ones I've listed below have been shown to have some proven efficacy, and I feel comfortable recommending them.

As with essential nutrients, the quality of nutraceuticals varies greatly. Many are produced overseas, where there is a complete lack of regulation. Therefore, I suggest that you look for products made in the United States whenever possible. And while their names sound quite benign, they actually can cause dangerous and adverse reactions when combined with prescription medication. Therefore, I also suggest that you talk with your doctor before taking any type of nutraceutical.

I also want to make it very clear that as far as I'm concerned, there is no one miracle supplement—vitamin, mineral, probiotic, fatty acid—that specifically targets belly fat or weight loss. Some researchers believe that supplementing with branched-chain amino acids such as leucine, isoleucine, and valine is an additional strategy to target troublesome fat, especially around the belly. These nutrients are the major building blocks for muscle tissue that play a critical role in regulating metabolism during exercise. When added to a solid nutritional and exercise program, these amino acids may help tap into the belly fat stores for energy. They may just give you that extra edge to get rid of your spare tire. But supplements are never enough: You have to do the hard work.

Bodybuilding magazines and websites also tout fat burners and muscle builders, both of which I believe are more hype than hard truth. They certainly don't do the work for you: You still need to get out and get sweaty in order to get the results that you are looking for. However, they are on the market, and if you are going to try one, I suggest that you try something that is as safe as possible.

HMB (hydroxy-methylbutyrate) is a relatively new ingredient that men are talking about because of its ability to burn fat and build muscle. It is a by-product of the amino acid leucine (the same one I just mentioned in terms of getting rid of belly fat) and is naturally found in only two types of food: catfish and grapefruit. It is also produced by the human body. HMB is an active ingredient in the popular Ensure product line: It is found in those drinks labeled "Revigor." Three other companies currently market the product as a dietary supplement.

Although it has not been widely studied, researchers claim that HMB enhances the gains in muscle strength and lean mass associated with resistance training by making proteins more available to the body, particularly after a workout. In doing so, HMB allows athletes to retain more protein in their system, resulting in increased energy levels and faster recovery. When we ingest extra amounts of HMB, it acts as a performance enhancer for such activities as weight lifting and sprinting. It boosts strength levels, enhances gains in muscle size and strength, and prevents postworkout muscle tissue breakdown. There have been no studies that contradict these findings.

How to Choose the Right Vitamins

Contrary to what most men believe, the supplement industry actually does have to follow some federal regulations, but not to the degree that the pharmaceutical industry does. At the same time, the FDA acknowledges that it has limited resources in relation to the supplement industry's size to adequately enforce regulations. They are supposed to regulate the manufacturing processes and marketing claims, focusing on labeling and product marketing (performed in conjunction with the FTC). For example, use of the term "Dietary Supplement" and claims of health benefits are regulated and defined by the FDA. Yet the terms "nutraceutical" and "functional food" are not regulated. New dietary ingredients don't have to be tested or registered before marketing. Perhaps most important, a supplement will be removed from the market shelves only after a product has proven to be unsafe.

When you are purchasing supplements, I recommend that you always look for high-quality, pharmaceutical-grade products. The supplement must be 99 percent pure and free of fillers, binders, and unknown substances, and pass a rigorous approval procedure by the United States Pharmacopeia (USP). Look for the words "USP approved" on labels or product information websites or pamphlets: This provides assurance to the consumer that the quality and purity of raw materials used in the manufacture of each supplement are of pharmaceutical grade and guarantees a certain standard of excellence.

There are several excellent-quality vitamin and mineral supplement lines available. My own nutraceuticals, which can be purchased on my website (www.drlife.com), are high-quality, pharmaceutical-grade products that I recommend. Dr. Kenneth H. Cooper has also created a line of excellent vitamin and mineral supplements. These products can be reviewed on his website, www.coopercomplete.com.

One of his products is called Cooper Complete Elite Athlete formulation. This is a vitamin/mineral supplement designed specifically for the high-endurance aerobic athletes, but I believe that it works equally well for anyone involved in high-intensity resistance training. It does lack calcium, so be sure you add a 1,000- or 1,200-milligram supplement to your regimen if you take this product. Less expensive products that have decent quality include Vita Smart Multi-Vitamins Men's and One A Day 50 Plus.

Remember: It's not enough just to buy them, you have to take your supplements. The most important rule about supplements is to take them consistently. They cannot help you if you let them sit in your cabinet. It sometimes takes several weeks to feel the effects or notice them working, but continue to take them to maximize your results.

Finally, vitamin and mineral supplementation alone won't get you all the thousands of micronutrients that are responsible for a multitude of health benefits. Even the best supplementation program must work with a balanced diet, such as the ones described in this book. This is why you need to make sure you eat plenty of nontropical fruits, vegetables, healthy fats, and high-quality, lean protein.

My Supplement Shopping List

Here are my suggestions for supplements that every active man needs in order to optimize his health and quality of life. You can adapt this based on your current health and your own doctor's recommendations.

It's best to split your daily supplements into a morning dose and an evening dose, because this allows your body to maintain a sufficient level of the water-soluble antioxidants needed to fight off free radicals. It really doesn't matter which ones you take in the morning or evening. Most comprehensive multivitamins/minerals are packaged in such a way that you take one serving in the morning and the other in the evening. I divide my fish oil into a morning serving and an evening serving. Melatonin should be taken at night, because it enhances sleep, and some of my patients think vitamin D_3 also helps them achieve a more restful sleep. As you read through the details for each of these supplement suggestions, you'll also see how they work together, and which should be taken at the same time.

1. Essential nutrient: Comprehensive multivitamin and mineral supplement

2. Essential nutrient: Essential fatty acids

3. Essential nutrient: Probiotic supplement

4. Essential nutrient: Vitamin D_3

5. Essential nutrient: Calcium

6. Nutraceutical: CoQ_{10}

7. Nutraceutical: Saw palmetto

8. Nutraceutical: Lycopene

9. Nutraceutical: Milk thistle

10. Nutraceutical: Pycnogenol/L-arginine

Comprehensive Multivitamin and Mineral Supplement

Every man needs a good multivitamin and mineral supplement every day: Consider these to be the most essential nutrients. Multivitamin capsules digest and metabolize faster than tablets. Make sure you pick one that has at least 100 percent of the Recommended Dietary Allowances (RDA) for thiamine (B_1), riboflavin (B_2), niacin (B_3), vitamins B_6, B_{12}, E, linoleic acid, and folic acid. You also need 2,000 milligrams of vitamin C, at least 400 IU of vitamin E, and at least 100 milligrams of magnesium. Your multivitamin should also contain at least 20 micrograms of vitamin K, as well as the minerals chromium, copper, selenium, and zinc (15 milligrams). If you are on a blood thinner (such as Coumadin), talk with your doctor about how much vitamin K you require.

Vitamin A toxicity can easily be avoided by simply taking beta-carotene, which your body converts to vitamin A. Beta-carotene doesn't cause bone loss, but too much beta-carotene may increase the risk of lung cancer if you are a smoker (which you shouldn't be, but you know that already). You don't need more than 15,000 IU daily of beta-carotene. The vitamin A in supplements can also come from retinol (often called vitamin A palmitate or acetate). To protect your bones, limit retinol to no more than 3,000 IU per day.

Essential Fatty Acids (EFAs)

My minimum recommendation for this essential nutrient is 300 to 500 milligrams daily. Purchase high-quality fish oil supplements that have the highest amount of eicosapentae-noic acid, EPA, and docosahexaenoic acid, DHA, per capsule, and keep them refrigerated. You need to take four one-gram capsules daily in order to create the best balance for your body. The content of high-quality fish oil should consist of at least 60 percent of both essential fatty acids (EPA and DHA) combined. The concentration of DHA should not be less than 18 percent, and a higher concentration is a signal of superior quality. EFAs show strong evidence for use as anti-inflammatories and in the promotion of overall health.

The highest-quality fish oil supplements are made in New Zealand and Norway. Oily fish found in these regions of the world are less contaminated by pollutants than similar fish found in other regions. Consequently, the oil obtained from them does not require as much purification. Always read the list of ingredients found on the bottle. If additives or preservatives have been added to increase shelf life, they might make the overall supplement less effective. Ultrarefined and ultrapurified fish oil products are better choices, because they typically are made from pharmaceutical-grade fish oil. Look for labels that indicate that the product has undergone "molecular distillation," which not only removes mercury and dioxin impurities but also balances out the concentration of other nutrients such as vitamins A and D, if present.

If you take cod liver oil (some men prefer this to fish oil capsules), be aware that it also contains vitamins A and D. Depending on how much cod liver oil you use and what other supplements you're taking, you could be getting too much of these vitamins. An alternative is devitaminized cod liver oil.

Because fish oil does not compensate for potential oxidative damage, it's also a good idea to increase your intake of vitamin E. I recommend that you take between 400 and

800 IU of vitamin E per day. While some fish oil capsules, as well as your multivitamin, may also contain some vitamin E, it may not be enough.

Probiotic Supplements

Probiotic supplements are considered essential nutrients and are available as capsules, powders, and tablets. I think it is prudent to include probiotics in your daily regimen, because they are thought to enhance fat metabolism, stimulate mineral absorption, improve GI function, and multiply "healthy" bacteria in the intestines. Choose one that is a blend of at least six "live" cultures and that is kept in a refrigerated case, and make sure to keep them refrigerated at home. Follow the manufacturer's recommended dosing on the label, since dosage can differ depending on the probiotic source.

Vitamin D$_3$

Vitamin D is really not a vitamin at all: It's a hormone. Yet it is still considered an essential nutrient in my book. Adequate vitamin D levels can protect you against cancer, infections, and premature aging. Vitamin D helps your body absorb calcium and is vital for skeletal development/health and prevention of osteoporosis. Vitamin D deficiency/insufficiency is also a risk factor for cardiovascular disease, hypertension, and type 2 diabetes. A June 2008 study reported that vitamin D deficiency gives men a 2.5 times higher risk for a heart attack. It also found that men with intermediate vitamin D levels demonstrated a 60 percent increased myocardial infarction risk. For all of these reasons, I believe that it is critical that every man get enough D.

Most men who work indoors have insufficient or deficient levels of vitamin D, because it is mostly (90 percent) manufactured in our skin when we are exposed to sunlight. Eating vitamin D–rich foods cannot solve the problem alone. If you live in the northern third of the United States, Canada, or Alaska, you're probably not getting enough vitamin D during the winter months. This, combined with the fact that most winter activity is limited to the indoors, results in many men having very little sun exposure.

Vitamin D supplementation is particularly important for overweight African-

American men. African-Americans have multiple risk factors for cardiovascular disease. According to Ryan A. Harris, Ph.D., assistant professor at the Georgia Prevention Institute at Georgia Health Sciences University, African-Americans are more likely than people of other races to develop type 2 diabetes, and when they develop high blood pressure it tends to be more severe as compared to other groups. African-Americans also have a greater risk of developing vitamin D deficiency, because their skin pigmentation inhibits the skin cells' ability to produce vitamin D in response to exposure to sunlight.

A blood test for 25-hydroxy-vitamin D is the best way to determine your status. Levels less than 30 ng/mL are considered a deficiency state. Optimal levels are 60 to 90 ng/mL. Most of my patients need to take 5,000 IU to 10,000 IU daily to achieve these levels, which is significantly less than what is offered in even the best multivitamin. Choose a supplement containing cholecalciferol (D_3), and make sure to talk to your doctor about vitamin D supplementation if you are currently taking antiseizure medications.

Calcium

Calcium is the most abundant mineral in the body. It is naturally found in some foods and is added to others, such as milk products. The safest and most effective source of calcium for strong bones and overall health is your diet, and many of the foods highlighted in my diet are high in calcium, including yogurt, tofu, almonds, kale, and broccoli. If you follow this diet strictly and make sure you are eating these foods as I recommend them, you don't have to further supplement with calcium. However, many American men do not consume enough foods to get the recommended intakes of this essential mineral, and they may therefore require a calcium dietary supplement or may need to take a daily antacid, such as Tums.

Calcium is required for muscle contraction, blood vessel expansion and contraction, secretion of hormones and enzymes, and transmitting impulses throughout the nervous system. The body strives to maintain constant concentrations of calcium in blood, muscle, and intercellular fluids. When our intake of calcium is low, the body willfully pulls calcium from bones in order to maintain critical concentrations. Then, as we age, our weakened bones can break down due to calcium loss, resulting in osteoporosis.

Calcium requires its own set of pills, because you need 1,000 to 1,200 milligrams daily, which is far less than what is available in a typical multivitamin. The two main forms of calcium found in supplements are calcium carbonate and calcium citrate. Calcium carbonate is more commonly available and is both inexpensive and convenient. Both the carbonate and citrate forms are similarly well absorbed, but men taking medications such as Pepcid that reduce levels of stomach acid can absorb calcium citrate more easily.

Coenzyme Q_{10}

Coenzyme Q_{10} is one nutraceutical that I fully stand behind. It is actually a vitaminlike chemical that is found in practically all the cells in the body, especially the heart. It has antioxidant properties, and the body uses it to generate ATP, the cellular storage unit of energy. Coenzyme Q_{10} levels start declining after the age of 20. Low levels of CoQ_{10} are thought to interfere with energy production pathways in our body.

The potential benefits of taking CoQ_{10} include antioxidant activity, prevention of age-related macular degeneration, enhancing athletic performance, improved immune function, prevention of heart disease, and slowing the aging process. Any man who is taking a statin drug to control cholesterol levels must take extra Coenzyme Q_{10} because statins deplete CoQ_{10} from skeletal and cardiac muscle. The recommended dose of Coenzyme Q_{10} is 100 milligrams if you are not on a statin and 200 milligrams daily if you are on a statin. Choose the form of CoQ_{10} called ubiquinol, which is the electron-rich form of this supplement and is used more efficiently by our bodies.

Saw Palmetto

Saw palmetto is another proven nutraceutical that is used mainly for relieving urinary symptoms associated with an enlarged prostate gland (benign prostatic hyperplasia, or BPH), such as frequent nighttime urination. Several small studies suggest that saw palmetto may be effective for treating BPH symptoms. However, a 2009 review of the research concluded that saw palmetto has not been shown to be more effective than a placebo for this use.

My experience is mixed; I believe it has significantly helped reduce the frequency and the number of times I have to get up at night. Others feel it hasn't helped them much. I think it's worthwhile to give it a try, since it is well tolerated by most men. Look for a supplement that is standardized to contain 85 to 95 percent fatty acids and sterols. Recommended dose is 160 milligrams twice a day.

Lycopene

Lycopene is a phytochemical nutraceutical that creates the bright red pigment found in tomatoes and other red fruits and vegetables, such as watermelons and papayas (but not strawberries or cherries). Research indicates that men who get more lycopene in their diet have a reduced risk of prostate cancer. Other research suggests lycopene supplementation inhibits progression of benign prostatic hyperplasia. It also has beneficial antioxidant effects.

I think it is prudent to take 20 milligrams daily of this nutrient. Compare this dosage to the ingredients in your multivitamin to ensure that you are covered: Many multis include lycopene as well. It is better absorbed when taken with a fatty acid, so make sure to take it at the same time as your fish oil supplements.

Milk Thistle

The seeds of the milk thistle have been used for over 2,000 years to treat chronic liver disease and protect the liver against toxins. It may also be useful in the prevention and treatment of prostate cancer. Look for a standardized extract of this nutraceutical that contains 70 percent silymarin at the dose of 200 milligrams twice a day.

Pycnogenol/L-arginine

Great sex requires a strong erection, which relies on the relaxation of the cavernous smooth muscle and dilation of blood vessels, which are triggered by the chemical nitric oxide (NO). Pycnogenol, a natural plant extract from the bark of the maritime pine tree, increases the production of your own nitric oxide. When pycnogenol is combined with L-arginine, this nutraceutical has been shown to produce a significant improvement in sexual function in men with erectile dysfunction (ED), without any side effects. The best dose is 40 milligrams of pycnogenol, two times a day, and two grams of L-arginine once a day. I have personally used this combination of supplements and can attest to its effectiveness for men with or without ED.

CHAPTER 13

Keep Moving Forward: Week 9 and Beyond

- -

Whether you've completed the entire eight-week program or are just ready to begin, congratulate yourself for taking control of your body and your overall health. Just by reading this book you've demonstrated your commitment to your future, and that is always the first step to making lasting change.

As I've said before, you are not going to see an overnight transformation, so don't expect one. It took me 19 weeks of grueling work to reach my first set of fat-loss goals when I was 59, and another 16 years to keep my body in top shape, and even looking better. Every day is a challenge, but one that I embrace. If you are up for staying the course, I know that you will meet your goals as well and join me in feeling younger every year. There are no limits to the success you can reach: At age 74 I was honored to be chosen by *Men's Fitness* magazine as one of the 25 Fittest Guys of 2012, and I was two to three times older than the other 24. Imagine what's in store for you.

Get Ready for the Life Plan

- -

Once you have the food program under your belt and have considered the necessary testing for hormone therapies, the last piece of the fat-loss puzzle is exercise. If you have been incorporating the walking suggestions, I'm sure you have already noticed how good a little exercise makes you feel. But what you might not know is how good it really is for you.

In terms of fat loss, exercise is by far the best way to maximize a caloric deficit, because it does not trigger the starvation response, it increases your metabolic rate, it increases all of the fat-burning enzymes and hormones, it targets body fat rather than muscle tissue for energy sources, and it increases the sensitivity of all cells to insulin so that carbohydrates are burned for energy and stored as glycogen rather than being stored as body fat. On top of this, exercise helps you create more muscle mass as you are trimming down your body fat. This is important because you need muscle to keep your metabolism running. The more muscle or lean body mass you have, the greater the number of calories you will burn throughout the day and the better you will feel. Trust me, plenty of muscle mass is a sure-fire way to avoid getting old as you age.

One of the added benefits of exercise is that it actually makes you feel like eating less. In a 2013 article in the *International Journal of Obesity*, researchers at the University of Western Australia found that strenuous exercise seems to dull the urge to eat afterward more than easier workouts. The exercise programs I lay out in my other two books feature strenuous interval-training sessions that match the results seen in these studies, which found that intense exercise leads to a short-term suppression of food intake.

The food plan described in this book is really the cornerstone to my entire program. Without it, even the best exercise plan and perfect hormone levels won't change the way your belly looks. A good exercise program is easy to put together and stick with, but it becomes even more effective once you get your diet in line. I've found that once my patients begin to lose body fat on the Life Plan Diet, they are not only more motivated to exercise, they actually have more energy to exercise. Both of these conditions allow them to see better and faster results. Just as with hormone therapies, exercise alone is not going to get you the results you are looking for: It's the combination that makes the program super effective.

For example, the typical 25- to 35-year-old guy I see working out at my gym is holding on to more than 25 percent body fat, mostly in his belly. These men aren't just sitting around: They're training hard, but they're not making any gains when it comes to the amount of muscle they have or lowering their percent body fat. The reason is that they haven't changed their diet. They may be getting stronger, but their belly isn't changing at all. I'm guessing that they believe that they can train hard and then eat and drink whatever they want.

One of these guys will eventually come up and ask me what my secret is. When I tell them about the diet, and how simple it is to stay with it, they're amazed. Then, when they try it out, I can see for myself how quickly those stubborn pounds start coming off them. Once they switch over and start doing the Life Plan Diet the way I do, even they can't believe the results.

My previous books, *The Life Plan* and *Mastering the Life Plan*, lay out exactly what a well-rounded exercise program should look like. Men need to do a combination of cardiovascular exercise, resistance or weight training, and flexibility/stretching in order to get the most benefit. These exercises have been calibrated to perfectly complement the diet. The foods you'll eat will support your workouts, and your workouts will continue to boost your metabolism, which is being fueled by the nutrient-rich foods on the diet. The foods you've been introduced to will also help strengthen your bones and muscles, which further support a more vigorous exercise program.

While this book is all about reducing belly fat, there really is no one exercise that accomplishes that mission. Sit-ups, crunches, and other abdominal exercises will strengthen your core muscles and help you lose some overall fat, but they don't specifically target belly fat. In other words, you can't spot-reduce. The only way to lose belly fat (or any kind of fat) is through the combination of dieting and exercise, and you'll see real fat loss occurring all over your body. Aerobic exercises, such as running, swimming, cycling, and tennis, are some of the best ways to help reduce body fat. I ride an exercise bike while I'm watching action movies to really tap into my maximum fat-burning potential. And I've got to tell you, when I combine the cardio with the right diet I can see and feel the changes in my body daily as the fat burns away.

If I've been able to teach you one lesson that goes beyond the kitchen table, it's that you're never too old or too out of shape to achieve real change to your health. Following a new eating plan looks simple, but I know that sticking with it for the long haul will be one of the hardest things that you are ever going to do. I know that you can take this challenge on and make it your own. Just remember what Diana Nyad said when she successfully swam from Havana to Miami in 2013, at age 64: "Never give up! You're never too old to chase your dream!"

The Life Plan Diet Food Journal

Y ou now have all the information you need to master the Life Plan Diet. The rest is up to you. Can you motivate yourself off the couch and into the gym? Can you find the time in even the busiest days to make change happen? For me, once I started there was no going back. I made a commitment to myself and I'm proud to say that 16 years later I still feel better every year than the year before. So for me, the choice is obvious. As I'm sure it will be for you.

I'm much better at sticking to a diet and exercise program if I write down every day exactly what I've accomplished. This works for me on several levels. First, it makes me accountable for everything that I put into my mouth. I then have a record to refer to so that I can track my success and be able to see why some weeks were more effective than others. Tracking my progress also provides a sense of satisfaction at the end of each day when I recognize that I was able to stay on track.

You can photocopy these pages or download them from my website, www.drlife.com. Put a week's worth of sheets in a binder or fold them in your wallet, and bring them with you wherever you go. You can also keep this information on your smartphone or iPad. I like to fill in the information as I go throughout the day, instead of trying to remember before bedtime what I ate or which exercises I performed. And by recording my meals right after

I eat them, I can see if I need to make small adjustments later on in the day. For example, if I had to eat breakfast out of the house, and the omelet I ordered at the restaurant was made with three eggs instead of two, I can choose a lower-calorie snack during the day to compensate.

It's crucial to stick with this program for the full twelve weeks. It generally takes that long just for your brain to create new habits and your body to get into the swing of clean eating. By then you will see significant changes to your physique.

The Life Plan Food Journal

After each meal, write down exactly what you ate. Also include the time that you ate and your level of hunger 20 minutes after eating, ranking it on a scale from 1 to 10. This is a good way of tracking your satiety, which can assist you in learning how to eat based upon hunger and timing rather than habit. Record how much water you drank during and previous to each meal so that you can add the amounts to see if you are meeting your goal. Finally, you can also check off if you took your supplements each day, and list weekly which ones you are taking.

Week #	Monday	Tuesday	Wednesday	Thursday	Friday	Saturday	Sunday
MEAL #1 Type: Time: Hunger level: oz of water:							
MEAL #2 Type: Time: Hunger level: oz of water:							
MEAL #3 Type: Time: Hunger level: oz of water:							
MEAL #4 Type: Time: Hunger level: oz of water:							
MEAL #5 Type: Time: Hunger level: oz of water:							
MEAL #6 Type: Time: Hunger level: oz of water:							
Supplements taken:							

After you have kept your workout and nutrition logs for a few weeks you can begin to analyze the information you have gathered. Try to be very objective when reading your logs and ask yourself the following questions:

1. Am I progressing? Am I losing weight and generally feeling better about the way I look and feel?

2. Are my clothes fitting differently? Is my waistline decreasing?

3. Am I tired after exercise? Am I working at my highest capability?

4. Am I taking my supplements? Am I skipping days, or maintaining consistency?

5. Am I sleeping better at night? Do I feel rested when I wake up in the morning, and do I go to sleep easily at night? Do I feel energized throughout the day, or sluggish?

6. Am I eating the right amount of balanced meals? Am I on track to reach my goals?

7. Am I drinking enough water?

Acknowledgments

This book would not have been possible without the love and support of my wife, Annie. I consider myself incredibly fortunate that she entered my life when she did, and she continues to provide me with the incentives I need to achieve optimal health. I'm especially thankful for all of the great recipes she has provided for my books.

I would also like to thank my agent, Carol Mann, and all the folks at Atria Books. Sarah Durand and Judith Curr support my vision, and their entire team has been tremendous to work with.

My writer, Pam Liflander, continues to help me get my thoughts and beliefs on paper, and then organize and craft all of them into words that perfectly describe what men need to know to stay healthy, lose weight, and avoid feeling old.

I'd like to thank Joey Carson for all of his support and friendship. Dr. Phil McGraw and his son, Jay, have been huge supporters of my mission. Lauren Tancredi helps keep me organized and on track. Mike Starks, founder and CEO of Personal Trainer Food, has played an important new role in my understanding of the fasting aspect of this new program. Jason Ellis, my photographer, has done an outstanding job helping me look my best on this new book cover.

Amy Doneen, MSN, ARNP, and Brad Bale, MD, creators of the Bale/Doneen Method for preventing heart attacks and strokes, continue to assist with my own heart health as well as the health of my patients. I would also like to thank my friends at Cenegenics for supporting my mission to improve men's health everywhere.

I would like to thank Dr. Max Sawaf, founder of Wellness Wave, for his encouragement and friendship. I am so impressed with his team that I have moved my medical practice to Wellness Wave in Beverly Hills.

Finally, none of this would have been possible if it weren't for the pioneering work of the late Alan P. Mintz, MD, the "Father of Age Management Medicine." We all miss him very much.

Resources

Siebold, Steve, *Die Fat or Get Tough: 101 Differences In Thinking Between Fat People and Fit People* (London House Press, 2010).

Carmona, Richard, *Canyon Ranch: 30 Days to a Better Brain* (Atria Books, 2013).

References

Chapter 1

Litwin, S. E. Good Fat, Bad Fat: The Increasingly Complex Interplay of Adipose Tissue and the Cardiovascular System. *J. Am. Coll. Cardiol.* 2013; 62(2):136–37. doi:10.1016/j.jacc.2013.04.028.

http://www.virtualmedicalcentre.com/health-investigation/assessing-central-obesity-waist-to-hip -ratio/73.

Thomson, C., Clark, S., and Jr., C. C. (2003). Body Mass Index and Asthma Severity Among Adults Presenting to the Emergency Department. *Chest Journal.* 2003, 124(3), 795–802.

Chapter 2

Christensen. K., M.D., Thinggaard, M., M.Sc., Oksuzyan, A., M.D., Steenstrup, T., Ph.D., Andersen-Ranberg, K., M.D., Jeune, B., M.D., McGue, M., Ph.D., Vaupel, J., Ph.D. Physical and cognitive functioning of people older than 90 years: A comparison of two Danish cohorts born 10 years apart. *The Lancet.* 2013, July 11, DOI: 10.1016/S0140-6736(13)60777-1.

Matthews, F., Ph.D., Arthur, A., Ph.D., Barnes, L., RGN, Bond, J., BA, Jagger, C., Ph.D., Robinson, L., M.D., Brayne, C., M.D. A two-decade comparison of prevalence of dementia in individuals aged 65 years and older from three geographical areas of England: Results of the Cognitive Function and Ageing Study I and II. *The Lancet.* 2013, July 17, DOI: 10.1016/S0140-6736(13)61570-6.

Chapter 3

Average waist circumference for men: http://www.cdc.gov/nchs/fastats/bodymeas.htm.

Browning, Lucy M., et al. A systematic review of waist-to-height ratio as a screening tool for the prediction of cardiovascular disease and diabetes: 05 could be a suitable global boundary value. *Nutrition Research Reviews*. 2010, 23 (02): 247–69. doi:10.1017/S0954422410000144.

Christakis, N. A., and Fowler, J. H. The Spread of Obesity in a Large Social Network Over 32 Years. *N. Engl. J. Med*. 2007, July 26, 357(4):370–79.

Kolata, G. Find Yourself Packing it On? Blame Friends. *New York Times*. July 26, 2007.

Chapter 4

Markwald, R., Melanson, E., Smith, M., Higgins, J., Perreault, L., Eckel, R., and Wright, K. Jr. Impact of insufficient sleep on total daily energy expenditure, food intake, and weight gain. *PNAS*. 2013; March 11, doi:10.1073/pnas.1216951110.

Broussard, J., Ehrmann, D., Van Cauter, E., Tasali, E., Brady, M. Impaired Insulin Signaling in Human Adipocytes After Experimental Sleep Restriction: A Randomized, Crossover Study. *Annals of Internal Medicine*. 2012, Oct.;157(8):549–57.

Intermountain Medical Center. Routine periodic fasting is good for your health, and your heart, study suggests. *ScienceDaily*. May 20, 2011. Web. Aug. 28, 2013.

Horne, B. D., Muhlestein, J. B., Lappé, D. L., May, H. T., Carlquist, J. F., Galenko, O., Brunisholz, K. D., and Anderson, J. L. Randomized cross-over trial of short-term water-only fasting: Metabolic and cardiovascular consequences. *Nutr. Metab. Cardiovasc. Dis*. 2012, Dec. 7, pii: S0939-4753(12)00257-8. doi: 10.1016/j.numecd.2012.09.007.

Chapter 5

St-Onge, M.-P., Salinardi, T., Herron-Rubin, K., and Black, R. A. Weight-Loss Diet Including Coffee-Derived Mannooligosaccharides Enhances Adipose Tissue Loss in Overweight Men but Not Women. *Obesity*. 2011, n. pag.

Pal, S., Ellis, V., and Dhaliwal, S. Effects of Whey Protein Isolate on Body Composition, Lipids, Insulin and Glucose in Overweight and Obese Individuals. *British Journal of Nutrition*. 2010, 104.05: 716–23.

Chapter 6

Mozaffarian, D., Hao, T., Rimm, E. B., Willett, W. C., and Hu, F. B. Changes in diet and lifestyle and long-term weight gain in women and men. *N. Engl. J. Med*. 2011, June 23, 364(25):2392-2404. doi: 10.1056/NEJMoa1014296.

Chapter 7

Colberg, S. R., Zarrabi, L., Bennington, L., Nakave, A., Thomas Somma, C., and Sechrist, S. R. Postprandial walking is better for lowering the glycemic effect of dinner than pre-dinner exercise in type 2 diabetic individuals. *J. Am. Med. Dir. Assoc.* 2009, 10(6):394–97.

Chapter 8

Ludwig, D. S. Examining the Health Effects of Fructose. *JAMA*. 2013, 310(1):33–34. doi:10.1001/jama.2013.6562.

Chapter 12

Testosterone References

Kaplan, A. L., and Hu, J. C. Use of Testosterone Replacement Therapy in the United States and Its Effect on Subsequent Prostate Cancer Outcomes. *Urology*. 2013, 82:321–26.

Tartavoulle, T. M., and Porche, D. J. Low Testosterone. *The Journal for Nurse Practitioners—JNP*. 2012, November/December, (8) 10, 778–82.

Hackett, G. Testosterone Replacement Improves Sexual Function, Aging Male Symptom and Depression Scores in a Primary Care Population of Men with Type 2 Diabetes. doi:10.1016/j.jomh.2011.08.091.

Hackett, G., Nigel, C., and Deshpande, A. Testosterone Replacement Improves Sexual Function, Aging Male Symptom and Depression Scores in a Primary Care Population of Men with Type 2 Diabetes. doi:10.1016/j.jomh.2011.08.093.

Zitzmann, M. Practical aspects in the use of testosterone replacement therapy for the family physician. 2011, April, *JMH*, Vol. 8, Suppl. 1, 597–5121.

Yamaguchi, K., Ishikawa, T., Chiba, K., and Fujisawa, M. Assessment of possible effects for testosterone replacement therapy in men with symptomatic late-onset hypogonadism. *Andrologia*. 2010, 43, 52–56.

Giagulli, V. A., Triggiani, V., Corona, G., Carbone, D., Licchelli, B., Tafaro, E., Resta, F., Sabbà, C., Maggi, M., and Guastamacchia, M. Evidence-based Medicine Update on Testosterone Replacement Therapy (TRT) in Male Hypogonadism: Focus on New Formulations. *Current Pharmaceutical Design*. 2011(7), 1500–11.

Khera, M., et al. Improved Sexual Function with Testosterone Replacement Therapy in Hypogonadal Men: Real-World Data from the Testim Registry in the United States (TRiUS). *J. Sex. Med.* 2011, 8:3204–3213.

McGill, J., et al. Androgen deficiency in older men: Indications, advantages, and pitfalls of testosterone replacement therapy. *Cleveland Clinical Journal of Medicine*. 2012, November 11, (79) 11, 797–806.

Baer, J. T. Testosterone replacement therapy to improve health in older males. *The Nurse Practitioner*. 2012, August, (37) 8: 39–44.

Chahla, E. J., et al. Testosterone replacement therapy and cardiovascular risk factors Modification. *The Aging Male*. 2011, June, 14(2): 83–90.

Ramasamy, R., et al. Testosterone Replacement Therapy and Prostate Cancer. *Indian Journal of Urology.* 2012, April, (28) 2, 123–28.

van den Beld, A., de Jong, F., et al. Measures of Bioavailable Serum Testosterone and Estradiol and Their Relationships with Muscle Strength, Bone Density, and Body Composition in Elderly Men. *J. Clin. Endocrinol. Metab.* 2000, Vol. 85, No. 9, 3276–82.

Bross, R., Javanbakht, M., and Bhasin, S. Anabolic Interventions for Aging-Associated Sarcopenia. *J. Clin. Endocrinol. Metab.* 1999, Vol. 84, No. 10, 3420–30.

Tenover, J. S. Effects of testosterone supplementation in the aging male. *J. Clin. Endocrinol. Metab.* 1992, Oct., 75(4):1092–98.

Shalender, B., and Tenover, J. S. Age-Associated Sarcopenia—Issues in the Use of Testosterone as an Anabolic Agent in Older Men. *J. Clin. Endocrinol. Metab.* 1997, Vol. 82, No. 6, 1659–60.

Urban, R. J., Bodenbrug, Y. H., et al. Testosterone administration to elderly men increases skeletal muscle strength and protein synthesis. *Am. J. Physiol.* 1995, Nov. 269(5 Pt 1):E820-6.

Snyder, P. The effects of testosterone treatment on body composition and metabolism in middle-aged obese men. *Int. J. Obes. Relat. Metab. Disord.* 1992, Dec., 16(12):991–97.

Snyder P., Peachey, H., Hannoush, P., et al. Effect of Testosterone Treatment on Bone Mineral Density in Men Over 65 Years of Age. *J. Clin. Endocrinol. Metab.* 1999, Vol. 84, No. 6, 1966–72. 1999.

Marin, P., Holmang, S., Jonsson, L., Sjostrom, L., Kvist, H., et al. The effects of testosterone treatment on body composition and metabolism in middle-aged obese men. *Int. J. Obes. Relat. Metab. Disord.* 1992, Dec., 16(12):991–97.

Sundeep Khosla, L., Melton, J., III, and Elizabeth, J. Relationship of Serum Sex Steroid Levels and Bone Turnover Markers with Bone Mineral Density in Men and Women: A Key Role for Bioavailable Estrogen. *J. Clin. Endocrinol. Metab.* 1998, Vol. 83, No. 7, 2266–74.

Chute, G. Sex hormones and coronary artery disease. *Am. J. Med.* 1987, Nov., 83(5):853–59.

Khaw, K. T., and Barrett-Connor, E. Lower endogenous androgens predict central adiposity in men. *Ann. Epidemiol.* 1992, Sep., 2(5):675–82.

Khaw, K. T., and Barrett-Connor, E. Blood pressure and endogenous testosterone in men: An inverse relationship. *J. Hypertens.* 1988, April, 6(4):329–32.

Marin, P., Krotkiewski, M., and Bjorntorp, P. Androgen treatment of middle-aged, obese men: Effects on metabolism, muscle and adipose tissues. *Eur. J. Med.* 1992, Oct., 1(6):329–36.

Zmuda, J. M., Cauley, J. A., Kriska, A., Glynn, N. W., Gutai, J. P., and Kuller, L. H. Longitudinal relation between endogenous testosterone and cardiovascular disease risk factors in middle-aged men: A 13-year follow-up of former Multiple Risk Factor Intervention Trial participants. *Amer. Journal of Epidemiology,* 1997, Oct. 15, 146(8):609–17.

English, K. M., Mandour, O., Steeds, R. P., Diver, M. J., Jones, T. H., and Channer, K. S. Men with coronary artery disease have lower levels of androgens than men with normal coronary angiograms. *Eur. Heart J.* 2000, June, 21(11):890–94.

English, K. M., Steeds, R. P., Jones, T. H., Diver, M. J., and Channer, K. S. Low-dose transdermal testosterone therapy improves angina threshold in men with chronic stable angina: A randomized, double-blind, placebo-controlled study. *Circulation*. 2000, Oct. 17, 102(16):1906–11.

Wu, S. Z., and Weng, X. Z. Therapeutic effects of an androgenic preparation on myocardial ischemia and cardiac function in 62 elderly male coronary heart disease patients. *Chin. Med. J. (Engl.)*. 1993, June, 106(6):415–18.

Webb, C. M., Adamson, D. L., de Zeigler, D., and Collins, P. Effect of acute testosterone on myocardial ischemia in men with coronary artery disease. *Am. J. Cardiol*. 1999, Feb. 1, 83(3):437–39, A9.

Muller, M. Endogenous Sex Hormones and Cardiovascular Disease in Men. *J. Clin. Endocrinol. Metab*. 2003, Vol. 88, No. 11, 5076–86.

Muller, M., Grobbee, D. E., den Tonkelaar, I., Lamberts, S. W., and van der Schouw, Y. T. Endogenous sex hormones and metabolic syndrome in aging men. *J. Clin. Endocrinol. Metab*. 2005, May, 90(5):2618–23.

Rupprecht, R. Neuroactive steroids: Mechanisms of action and neuropsychopharmacological properties. *Psychoneuroendocrinology*. 2003, Feb., 28(2):139–68.

Moffat, S. D., et al. Free testosterone and risk for Alzheimer disease in older men. *Neurology*. 2004, Jan. 27, 62(2): 188–93.

Gouras, G. K., Xu, H., Gross, R. S., et al. Testosterone reduces neuronal secretion of Alzheimer's β-amyloid peptides. *Proc. Natl. Acad. Sci. USA*. 2000, 97: 1202–5.

Papasozomenos, S. Ch., and Shanavas, A. Testosterone prevents the heat shock-induced overactivation of glycogen synthase kinase-3 beta but not of cyclin-dependent kinase 5 and c-Jun NH2-terminal kinase and concomitantly abolishes hyperphosphorylation of tau: implications for Alzheimer's disease. *Proc. Natl. Acad. Sci. USA*. 2002, Feb. 5, 99(3):1140–45.

Gillett, M. J., Martins, R. N., Clarnette, R. M., Chubb, S. A., Bruce, D. G., and Yeap, B. B. Relationship between testosterone, sex hormone binding globulin and plasma amyloid beta peptide 40 in older men with subjective memory loss or dementia. *J. Alzheimers Dis*. 2003, Aug., 5(4):267–69.

Tan, R. S., and Pu, S. J. A pilot study on the effects of testosterone in hypogonadal aging male patients with Alzheimer's disease. *Aging Male*. 2003, Mar., 6(1):13–17.

Hogervorst, E., Combrinck, M., et al. Testosterone and gonadotropin levels in men with dementia. *Neuro. Endocrinol. Lett*. 2003, 24(3–4):203–8.

Hogervorst, E., Bandelow, S., Combrinck, M., and Smith, A. D. Low free testosterone is an independent risk factor for Alzheimer's disease. *Experimental Gerontology*. 2004, Nov.–Dec., 39(11–12):1633–39.

Paoletti, A. M., et al. Low androgenization index in elderly women and elderly men with Alzheimer's disease. *Neurology*. 2004, Jan. 27, 62(2):301–3.

Ramzi, R., Kaiser, F., and Morley, J. Outcomes of Long-Term Testosterone Replacement in Older Hypogonadal Males: A Retrospective Analysis. *J. Clin. Endocrinol. Metab*. 1997, Vol. 82, No. 11, 3793–96.

Kwan, M., Greenleaf, W. J., Mann, J., Crapo, L., and Davidson, J. M. The nature of androgen action on male sexuality: A combined laboratory–self-report study on hypogonadal men. *J. Clin. Endocrinol. Metab*. 1983, Vol. 57, 557–62.

Skakkebaek, N. E., Bancroft, J., Davidson, D. W., and Warner, P. Androgen replacement with oral testosterone undecenoate in hypogonadal men: A double blind controlled study. *Clin. Endocrinol. (Oxf.).* 1981, 14:49–61.

O'Carroll, R., and Bancroft, J. Testosterone therapy for low sexual interest and erectile dysfunction in men: A controlled study. *Br. J. Psychiatry.* 1984, Aug., 145:146–51.

Ebert, T., Jockenhovel, F., Morales, A., et al. The current status of therapy for symptomatic late-onset hypogonadism with transdermal testosterone gel. *Eur. Urol.* 2005, Feb., 47(2):137–46.

Carani, C., Zini, D., Baldini, A., et al. Effects of androgen treatment in impotent men with normal and low levels of free testosterone. *Arch. Sex. Behav.* 1990, June, 19(3):223–34.

Jain, J. Urol Effect of exogenous testosterone on prostate volume, serum and semen prostate specific antigen levels in healthy young men. *J. Urol.* 1998, Feb., 159(2):441–43.

Cooper, C. S., Perry, P. J., and Sparks, et al. Effect of exogenous testosterone on prostate volume, serum and semen prostate specific antigen levels in healthy young men. *J. Urol.* 1998, Feb., 159(2):441–43.

Margolese, H. C. The male menopause and mood: testosterone decline and depression in the aging male—is there a link? *J. Geriatr. Psychiatry Neurol.* 2000, Summer, 13(2):93–101.

Morley, J. E. Testosterone replacement and the physiologic aspects of aging in men. *Mayo Clin. Proc.* 2000, Jan., 75 Suppl:S83–7.

Basaria, S., Wahlstrom, J., and Dobs, A. Anabolic-Androgenic Steroid Therapy in the Treatment of Chronic Diseases. *J. Clin. Endocrinol. Metab.* 2001, Vol. 86, No. 11, 5108–17.

Hoffman, M. A., DeWolf, W. C., and Morgentaler, A. Is low serum free testosterone a marker for high grade prostate cancer? *J. Urol.* 2000, March, 163(3):824–27.

Asbell, S. O., Raimane, K. C., Montesano, A. T., Zeitzer, K. L., Asbell, M. D., and Vijayakumar, S. Prostate-specific antigen and androgens in African-American and white normal subjects and prostate cancer patients. *J. Natl. Med. Assoc.* 2000, Sep., 92(9):445–49.

Rhoden, E. L., and Morgentaler, A. Risks of testosterone-replacement therapy and recommendations for monitoring, *N. Engl. J. Med.* 2004, Jan. 29, 350(5):482–92.

Carter, H. B., et al. Longitudinal evaluation of serum androgen levels in men with and without prostate cancer. *Prostate.* 1995, July, 27(1):25–31.

Conway, H. J. Randomized clinical trial of testosterone replacement therapy in hypogonadal men. *Int. J. Androl.* 1988, Aug., 11(4):247–64.

Pugh, P., Jones, T. H., and Channer, K. Acute Haemodynamic effects of testosterone in men with chronic heart failure. *European Heart Journal.* 2003, 24, 909–15.

Caminiti, G., Volterrani, M., et al. Effect of Long-Acting Testosterone Treatment on Function Exercise Capacity, Skeletal Muscle Performance, Insulin Resistance, and Baroreflex Sensitivity in Elderly Patients with Chronic Heart Failure: A Double-Blind, Placebo Controlled, Randomized Study. *J. Am. Coll. Cardiol.* 2009, 54; 919–27.

Malkin, C., et al. Testosterone Therapy in men with moderate severity heart failure: A double-blind randomized placebo controlled trial. *European Heart Journal.* 2006, 24, 54–64.

Hyde, Z., et al. Low Free Testosterone Predicts Frailty in Older Men: The Health in Men Study. *J. Clin. Endocrinol. Metab.* 2001, April 21, (95) 7, 3165–72.

Menke, A., et al. Sex Steroid Hormone Concentrations and Risk of Death in US Men. *American Journal of Epidemiology.* 2009, (171) 5, 583–92.

Srinivas-Shankar, U. Effects of Testosterone on Muscle Strength, Physical Function, Body Composition and Quality of Life in Intermediate-Frail and Frail Elderly Men: A Randomized, Double-Blind, Placebo-Controlled Study. *J. Clin. Endocrinol. Metab.* 2010, (95) 2, 639–50.

Sattler, F. R., et al. Testosterone and Growth Hormone Improve Body Composition and Muscle Performance in Older Men. *J. Clin. Endocrinol. Metab.* 2009, (94) 6, 1991–2001.

Maggio, M., et al. Relationship Between Low Levels of Anabolic Hormones and 6-Year Mortality Rate in Older Men. *Archives of Internal Medicine.* 2007, (167) 20 2249–54.

Wu, F., et al. Identification of Late-Onset Hypogonadism in Middle-Aged and Elderly Men. *N. Engl. J. Med.* 2010, (363): 123–35.

Finkelstein, J. S., et al. Gonadal Steroids and Body composition, Strength, and Sexual Function in Men. *N. Engl. J. Med.* 2013, Sep. 12, (369)11, 1011–22.

Growth Hormone References

Rasmussen, M. Obesity, growth hormone and weight loss. *Molecular and Cellular Endocrinology.* 2010, 316, 147–53.

Lyle, G. Human Growth Hormone and Anti-Aging: Safety and Efficacy Report. *Plastic and Reconstructive Surgery.* 2002, November, 110, No. 6, 1585–89.

Cardona, B., and Neilson, B. The logics of human growth hormone and the predicaments of old age. *Continuum: Journal of Media & Cultural Studies.* 2011, December, 25, No. 6, 857–71.

López, B. Creating fear: The social construction of human Growth Hormone as a dangerous doping drug. *International Review for the Sociology of Sport.* 2012, 48(2), 220–37.

Society for Endocrinology, Practice and Policy, Growth Hormone. http://www.endocrinology.org/policy /docs/gh.html.

Fowelin, J., Attrall, S., Lager, I., Bengtsson, B.-Å. Effects of treatment with recombinant human growth hormone on insulin sensitivity and glucose metabolism in adults with growth hormone deficiency. *Metabolism.* 1993, 42, 1443–47.

Johansson, J.-Q., Landin, K., Tengboru, L., Rosén, T., Bengtsson, B.-Å. High fibrinogen and plasminogen activator inhibitor activity in growth hormone deficient adults. *Arterioscler. Thromb.* 1994, 14, 434–37.

Markussis, V., Beshyah, S. A., Fischer, C., Sharp, P., Nicolaides, A. N., and Johnson, D. G. Detection of premature atherosclerosis by high resolution ultrasonography in symptom-free hypopituitary adults. *Lancet.* 1992, 340, 1188–92.

Capaldo, B., Patti, L., Oliverio, U., Longobardi, S., Pardo, F., Vitali, F., Fazio, S., di Reller, F., Bindi, B., Lombardi, G., and Sacca, L. Increased arterial intimi-media thickness in childhood onset growth hormone deficiency. *J. Clin. Endocrinol. Metab.* 1997, 82, 1378–81.

Rosén, T., and Bengtsson, B.-Å. Premature mortality due to cardiovascular disease in hypopituitarism. *Lancet*. 1990, 336, 285–88.

Bülow, B., Hacrmar, L., Mikoczy, Z., Nordström, C. H., and Erfurth, E. M. Increased cerebrovascular mortality in patient with hypopituitarism. *Clinical Endocrinology*. 1997, 46, 75–81.

American Association of Clinical Endocrinologist Medical Guidelines for Clinical Practice for Growth Hormone Use in Growth Hormone Deficient Adults and Transition Patients—October 2009 Update. *Endocrine Practice*. 2009, 15(2), 1.

Murray, R., Bidlingmaier, M., Strasburger, C., and Shalet, S. The Diagnosis of Partial Growth Hormone Deficiency in Adults with a Putative Insult to the Hypothalamo-Pituitary Axis. *J. Clin. Endocrinol. Metab.* 2007, 92(5):1705–9.

Consensus Statement. Consensus guidelines for the diagnosis and treatment of adults with GH deficiency II: A statement of the GH Research Society in association with the European Society for Pediatric Endocrinology, Lawson Wilkins Society, European Society of Endocrinology, Japan Endocrine Society, and Endocrine Society of Australia. *European Journal of Endocrinology*. 2007, 157, 695–700.

Murray, R. D., and Shalet, S. M. Insulin Sensitivity Is Impaired in Adults with Varying Degrees of GH Deficiency. *Clin. Endocrinol.* 2005, Feb., 62(2):182–88.

Murray, R. D., Adams, J. E., and Shalet, S. M. Adults with Partial Growth Hormone Deficiency Have an Adverse Body Composition. *J. Clin. Endocrinol. Metab.* 2004, Apr., 89(4):1586–91.

Colao, A., Cerbone, G., Pivonello, R., Aimaretti, G., Loche, S., Di Somma, C., Faggiano, A., Corneli, G., Ghigo, E., and Lombardi, G. The Growth Hormone (GH) Response to the Arginine Plus GH-Releasing Hormone Test Is Correlated to the Severity of Lipid Profile Abnormalities in Adult Patients with GH Deficiency. *J. Clin. Endocrinol. Metab.* 1999, Apr., 84(4):1277–82.

Colao, A., Di Somma, C., Spiezia, S., Rota, F., Pivonello, R., Savastano, S., and Lombardi, G. The Natural History of Partial Growth Hormone Deficiency in Adults: A prospective study on the cardiovascular risk and atherosclerosis. *J. Clin. Endocrinol. Metab.* 2006, June, 91(6):2191–2200.

Pandian, R., and Nakamoto, J. Rational use of the laboratory for childhood and adult growth hormone deficiency. *Clin. Lab. Med.* 2004, Mar., 24(1):141–74.

Vestergaard, P., and Hoeck, H. C. Reproducibility of growth hormone and cortisol responses to the insulin tolerance test and the short ACTH test in normal adults. *Horm. Metab. Res.* 1997, Mar., 29(3): 106–10.

Hoeck, H. C. Test of growth hormone secretion in adults: Poor reproducibility of the insulin tolerance test. *Eur. J. Endocrinol.* 1995, Sep. 1, 133(3): 305–12.

Biller, B. Sensitivity and Specificity of Six Tests for the Diagnosis of Adult GH Deficiency. *J. Clin. Endocrinol. Metab.* 2002, May, 87(5):2067–79.

Hoeck, H. C. Diagnosis of growth hormone (GH) deficiency in adults with hypothalamic-pituitary disorders: Comparison of test results using pyridostigmine plus GH-releasing hormone (GHRH), clonidine plus GHRH, and insulin-induced hypoglycemia as GH secretagogues. *J. Clin. Endocrinol. Metab.* 2000, Apr., 85(4):1467–72.

Boquete, H. R. Evaluation of diagnostic accuracy of insulin-like growth factor (IGF)-I and IGF-binding protein-3 in growth hormone-deficient children and adults using ROC plot analysis. *J. Clin. Endocrinol. Metab.* 2003, Oct., 88(10):4702–8.

Bonert, V. S. Body mass index determines evoked growth hormone (GH) responsiveness in normal healthy male subjects: Diagnostic caveat for adult GH deficiency. *J. Clin. Endocrinol. Metab.* 2004, July, 89(7):3397–3401.

Hartman, M. L., et al. Which patients do not require a GH stimulation test for the diagnosis of adult GH deficiency? *J. Clin. Endocrinol. Metab.* 2002, Feb., 87(2):477–85.

Carroll, et al. Growth hormone deficiency in adulthood and the effects of growth hormone replacement: A review. Growth Hormone Research Society Scientific Committee. *J. Clin. Endocrinol. Metab.* 1998, Feb., 83(2):382–95.

Franco, C. Growth hormone treatment reduces abdominal visceral fat in postmenopausal women with abdominal obesity: A 12-month placebo-controlled trial. *J. Clin. Endocrinol. Metab.* 2005, Mar. 1, 90(3): 1466–74.

Albert, S. Low-Dose Recombinant Human Growth Hormone as Adjuvant Therapy to Lifestyle Modifications in the Management of Obesity. *J. Clin. Endocrinol. Metab.* 2004, Feb.,Vol. 89, No. 2.

Johannsson, G. Growth Hormone Treatment of Abdominally Obese Men Reduces Abdominal Fat Mass, Improves Glucose and Lipoprotein Metabolism, and Reduces Diastolic Blood Pressure. *J. Clin. Endocrinol. Metab.* 1997, Vol. 82, No. 3, 727–34.

http://www.ghresearchsociety.org/bin/Default.asp.

Larsen, Kronnenberg, Melmed, and Polonsky (eds). *Williams Textbook of Endocrinology* (Saunders, 2003), Tenth Edition, Chapter 8, authored by Shlomo Melmed and David Kleinberg, summarizes Adult Somatotropin Deficiency in Table 8-20, p. 226, and they point out that IGF-1 levels may be "low or normal" in adult deficiency states.

Colao, A., et al. The National History of Partial Growth Hormone Deficiency in Adults: A Prospective Study on Cardiovascular Risk and Atherosclerosis. *J. Clin. Endocrinol. Metab.* 2006, June, Vol. 91, No. 6, 2191–2200.

Drake, W. M. Optimizing Growth Hormone Therapy in Adults and Children. *Endocr. Rev.* 2001, Aug. 1, 22(4): 425–50.

Mukherjee, A. Seeking the optimal target range for insulin-like growth factor I during the treatment of adult growth hormone disorders. *J. Clin. Endocrinol. Metab.* 2003, Dec., 88(12):5865–70.

Roubenof, R. Cytokines, insulin-like growth factor-1, sarcopenia, and mortality in very old community-dwelling men and women: The Framingham Heart Study. A*m. J. Med.* 2003, Oct. 15, 115(6): 429–35.

Cappola, A. Insulin-like growth factor I and interleukin-6 contribute synergistically to disability and mortality in older women. *J. Clin. Endocrinol. Metab.* 200, 3 May, 88(5):2019–25.

Laughlin, G. A., et al. The prospective association of serum insulin-like growth factor I (IGF-I) and IGF-binding protein-1 levels with all cause and cardiovascular disease mortality in older adults: The Rancho Bernardo Study. *J. Clin. Endocrinol. Metab.* 2004, Jan. 1, 89(1):114–20.

Gelato, M. Aging and Immune Function: A Possible Role for Growth Hormone. *Hormone Research.* 1996, 45:46–49.

Toogood, A. A., et al. Beyond the Somatopause: Growth Hormone Deficiency in Adults over the age of 60 years. *J. Clin. Endocrinol. Metab.* 1996, 82:460–65.

Young, A. Muscle Function in Old Age. *New Issue Neuroscience.* 1998, I:141–56.

Skeleton, D. A., et al. Strength, Power & Related Functional Ability of Healthy People Aged 60–89 years. *Aging People.* 199, 23:371–77.

Bohannon, R. W. Comfortable and maximum walking speed of adults aged 20–79 years: Reference Values and Determinants. *Age Ageing.* 1997, 26:15–19.

O'Connor, Ph.D. Thesis, Dublin, 1998.

Vahl, N., et al. Abdominal adiposity and physical fitness are major determinants of age associated decline in stimulated growth hormone secretion in healthy adults. *J. Clin. Endocrinol. Metab.* 1997, 816: 2209–15.

Savine, R., and Sonksen, P. Growth Hormone—Hormone Replacement for Somatopause. *Horm. Res.* 2000, 53(Suppl 3):37–41.

Conti, E., et al. Insulin-Like Growth Factor-1 as a Vascular Protective Factor. *Circulation.* 2004, 110, 2260–65.

Denti, L., et al. Insulin-like growth factor 1 as a predictor of ischemic stroke outcome in the elderly. *Am. J. Med.* 2004, Sep. 1, 117(5):312–17.

Juul, A., et al. Low serum insulin-like growth factor-1 is associated with increased risk of ischemic heart disease: A population-based case-control study. *Circulation.* 2002, 106:939–44.

Vasan, R. S., et al. Serum insulin-like growth factor-1 and risk for heart failure in elderly individuals without a previous myocardial infarction: The Framingham Heart Study. *Ann. Intern. Med.* 2003, 139:642–48.

Evaluation and Treatment of AGHD: An Endocrine Society Clinical Practice Guideline. *J. Clin. Endocrinol. Metab.* 2006, 91:1621–34.

Consensus Guideline for the Diagnosis and Treatment of Adults with Growth Hormone Deficiency II. *Endo.* 2007, 157: 695–700.

Melmed, S. Supplemental growth hormone in healthy adults: The endocrinologist's responsibility. *Nature Clinical Practice.* 2006, 2:119.

Critical evaluation of the safety of recombinant human growth hormone administration: Statement from the Growth Hormone Research Society. *J. Clin. Endocrinol. Metab.* 2001, 86:1868–70.

Bjorntorp, P. "Portal" adipose tissue as a generator of risk factors for cardiovascular disease and diabetes. *Arteriosclerosis.* 1990, 10:493–96.

Veldhuis, J. D. Neuroendocrine control of pulsatile growth hormone release in the human: relationship with gender: *Growth Hormone IGF-1 Res 8* (Suppl B).1998, 49–59.

Vahl, N., et al. Abdominal adiposity rather than age and sex predicts mass and regularity of GH secretion in healthy adults. *Am. J. Physiol.* 1997, 272:E1108–16.

Pasarica, M., et al. Effect of Growth Hormone on Body Composition and Visceral Adiposity in Middle-Aged Men with Visceral Obesity. *J. Clin. Endocrin. Metab.* 2007, 92:4265–70.

Beauregard, C., et al. Growth Hormone Decreases Visceral Fat and Improves Cardiovascular Risk Markers in Women with Hypopituitarism: A Randomized, Placebo-Controlled Study. *J. Clin. Endocrin. Metab.* First published ahead of print, 2008, April 1, as doi:10.1210/jc.2007–2371.

Simpson, H., et al. Growth hormone replacement therapy for adults: Into the new millennium. *Growth Horm. IGF Res.* 2002; 12:1–33.

de Boer, H., et al. Clinical aspects of growth hormone deficiency in adults. *Endocr. Rev.* 1995, 16:63–86.

Bengtsson, B.-Å., et al. Treatment of adults with growth hormone deficiency: Results of a 13-month placebo controlled cross over study. *Clin. Endocrinol. (Oxf.).* 1993, 76:309–17.

Snel, Y. E., et al. Magnetic resonance image-assessed adipose tissue and serum lipid and insulin concentrations in growth hormone deficient adults: Effects of growth hormone replacement. *Arterioscler. Thromb. Vasc. Biol.* 1995, 15:1543–48.

Hartman, M., et al. Growth Hormone Replacement Therapy in Adults with Growth Hormone Deficiency Improves Maximal Oxygen Consumption Independently of Dosing Regimen or Physical Activity. *J. Clin. Endocrin. Metab.* 2008, 93:125–30.

Kwan, A., and Hartman, M. IGF-1-1 measurements in the diagnosis of adult growth hormone deficiency. *Pituitary.* 2007, 10(2):151–57.

Clemmons, D. R., and Underwood, L. E. Nutritional regulation of IGF-1-1 and IGF-1 binding proteins. *Annu. Rev. Nutr.* 1991, 11:393–412.

Hartman, M. L. Physiological regulators of growth hormone secretion. In: Juul, A., and Jorgensen, J. O. L. (eds), *Growth Hormone in Adults*, Second Edition (Cambridge: Cambridge University Press, 2000), 3–53.

Baker, H. W., et al. Arginine-infusion test for growth-hormone secretion. *Lancet.* 1970, 2(7684):1193.

Juul, A. Serum levels of insulin-like growth factor I and its binding proteins in health and disease. *Growth Horm. IGF-1 Res.* 2003, 13:113–70.

Larsson, S. C., et al. Association of diet with serum insulin-like growth factor I in middle aged and elderly men. *Am. J. Clin. Nutr.* 2005, 81:1163–67.

Clasey, J. L., et al. Abdominal visceral fat and fasting insulin are important predictors of 24-hr GH release independent of age, gender, and other physiological factors. *J. Clin. Endocrinol. Metab.* 2001, 86(8):3845–52.

Rasmussen, M. H., et al. Massive weight loss restores 24-hr growth hormone release profiles and serum insulin-like growth factor-1 levels in obese subjects. *J. Clin. Endocrinol. Metab.* 1995, 80(4):1407–15.

Giustina, A., and Veldhuis, J. D. Pathophysiology of the neuroregulation of growth hormone secretion in experimental animals and the human. *Endocrin. Rev.* 1998, 19(6):717–97.

Felsing, N. E., et al. Effect of low and high intensity exercise on circulating growth hormone in men. *J. Clin. Endocrinol. Metab.* 1992, 75(1):157–62.

Weltman, A., et al. Endurance training amplifies the pulsatile release of growth hormone: Effects of training intensity. *J. Appl. Physiol.* 1992, 72(6):2188–96.

Weltman, A., et al. Relationship between age, percentage body fat, fitness and 24-hour growth hormone release in healthy young adults: Effect of gender. *J. Clin. Endocrinol. Metab.* 1994, 78:543–48.

Vahl, N., et al. Abdominal adiposity and physical fitness are major determinants of the age associated decline in stimulated GH secretion in healthy adults. *J. Clin. Endocrinol. Metab.* 1996, 81(6): 2209–15.

Yuen, K., et al. Is Lack of Recombinant Growth Hormone (GH)-Releasing Hormone in the United States a Setback or Time to Consider Glucagon Testing for Adult GH Deficiency? *J. Clin. Endocrinol. Metab.* 2009, 94: 2702–7.

Holt, R. Growth hormone: A potential treatment option in diabetes? *Diabetic Voice.* 2003, July, Vol. 48, Issue 2.

Cauter, E., et al. Age-related Changes in Slow Wave Sleep and REM Sleep and Relationship With Growth Hormone and Cortisol Levels in Healthy Men. *JAMA.* 2000, Aug. 16, 284, No. 7, 861–67.

Van Bunderen, C., et al. The Association of Serum Insulin-Like Growth Factor-I with Mortality, Cardiovascular Disease, and Cancer in the Elderly: A Population-Based Study. *J. Clin. Endocrinol. Metab.* 2010. (95) 9, 4449–54.

Popovic, V., et al. Serum Insulin-Like Growth Factor I (IGF-I), IGF-Binding Proteins 2 and 3 and the Risk for Development of Malignancies in Adults with Growth Hormone (GH) Deficiency Treated with GH: Data from KIMS (Pfizer International Metabolic Database). *J. Clin. Endocrinol. Metab.* 2010 (online).

Meinhardt, U., M.D., et al. The Effects of Growth Hormone on Body Composition and Physical Performance in Recreational Athletes: A Randomized Trial. *Annals of Internal Medicine.* 2010, May 4, (152) 9, 568–77.

Movérare-Skrtic, S., et al. Serum Insulin-Like Growth Factor-I Concentration Is Associated with Leukocyte Telomere Length in a Population-Based Cohort of Elderly Men. *J. Clin. Endocrinol. Metab.* 2009, Dec., (94) 12, 5078–84.

Makimura, H., et al. Reduced Growth Hormone Secretion Is Associated with Increased Carotid Intima-Media Thickness in Obesity. *J. Clin. Endocrinol. Metab.* 2009, (94) 12, 5131–38.

Colao, A., et al. Growth Hormone Treatment on Atherosclerosis: Results of a 5-Year Open, Prospective, Controlled Study in Male Patients with Severe Growth Hormone Deficiency. *J. Clin. Endocrinol. Metab.* 2008, (93) 9, 3416–24.

Colao, A., et al. The Natural History of Partial Growth Hormone Deficiency in Adults: A Prospective Study on Cardiovascular Risk and Atherosclerosis. *J. Clin. Endocrinol. Metab.* 2006, (91) 6, 2191–2200.

Colao, A., et al. Short-Term Effects of Growth Hormone (GH) Treatment or Deprivation on Cardiovascular Risk Parameters and Intima-Media Thickness at Carotid Arteries in Patients with Severe GH Deficiency. *J. Clin. Endocrinol. Metab.* 2005, (90)4, 2056–62.

Cittadini, A., et al. Growth Hormone Deficiency in Patients with Chronic Heart Failure and Beneficial Effects of Its Correction. *J. Clin. Endocrinol. Metab.* 2009, (94) 3329–36.

Fazio, S., et al. Effects of Growth Hormone on Exercise Capacity and Cardiopulmonary Performance in Patients with Chronic Heart Failure *J. Clin. Endocrinol. Metab.* 2007, (92) 11, 4218–23.

Le Corvoisier, P., et al. Cardiac Effects of Growth Hormone Treatment in Chronic Heart Failure: A Meta-Analysis. *J. Clin. Endocrinol. Metab.* 2007, (92) 1, 180–85.

Sattler, F. R., et al. Testosterone and Growth Hormone Improve Body Composition and Muscle Performance in Older Men. *J. Clin. Endocrinol. Metab.* 2009, (94) 6, 1991–2001.

Stoving, R. K., et al. Low Circulating Insulin-Like Growth Factor I Bioactivity in Elderly Men Is Associated with Increased Mortality. *J. Clin. Endocrinol. Metab.* 2008, (93) 7, 2515–22.

Savastano, S., et al. Growth Hormone Treatment Prevents Loss of Lean Mass after Bariatric Surgery in Morbidly Obese Patients: Results of a Pilot, Open, Prospective Randomized Controlled Study. *J. Clin. Endocrinol. Metab.* 2009, (94) 3, 817–26.

Chapter 13

Sim, A. Y., Wallman, K. E., Fairchild, T. J., and Guelfi, K. J. High-intensity intermittent exercise attenuates ad-libitum energy intake. *Int. J. Obes. (Lond.).* 2013, June 4, doi: 10.1038/ijo.2013.102.

Index

Page numbers in *italics* indicate locations of Annie's recipes

A

abdomen:
>of Life, 1, 5–6
>obesity and, 11, 13, 22, 24, 30
>and thinking like a lean and fit man, 52–53
>*see also* waist, waistline

abdominal muscles, 46, 114
>goals and, 41, 48–49
>six-pack, 5–6, 41, 48, 81

adipokines, 16

adrenal glands, 13, 202

advanced glycation end-products (AGEs), 18

African-Americans, 211–12

age, aging, 4, 27, 76, 108–10, 205, 219
>abdominal muscles and, 6
>belly fat and, 11, 14, 16, 30
>BMI and, 45
>body fat and, 42, 44
>brain and, 29–30, 34
>carbohydrate sensitivity and, 70
>cravings and, 51
>dietary fats and, 63
>exercise and, 218
>fitness and, 8, 50
>glycation and, 18

goals and, 41
hormones and, 25, 192–95, 198, 200, 202
inflammation and, 20
insulin and, 17
and letters from Life's patients, 47, 78–79, 89, 120–21, 125, 136, 148, 159
of Life, 1–3, 5, 7, 21, 31–32, 42, 53, 115, 217
metabolic syndrome and, 21
metabolism and, 58
and shortness of breath, 22
small meals and, 75
stress and, 33
supplements and, 204, 211–13
weight gain and, 42–43

alcohol, 35, 37–39, 58, 114
>avoidance of, 81–83
>glycemic index of, 68
>Life's consumption of, 2, 7, 32, 39, 82
>parties and, 107
>restaurants and, 106
>sexuality and, 25, 83
>stress and, 32–33
>testosterone and, 198
>and thinking like a lean and fit man, 51–53
>weight loss goals and, 49

almonds, 140, 212
>chocolate almond protein shake, *186*
>JumpStart Diet and, 118, 122
>pork chops with cherries and almonds, *185*
>recipes and, 132, 145, 166, 168, 175, 185–86, 188
>shopping list and, 94, 99

alpha-linolenic acid (ALA), 65

Alzheimer's disease, 15, 50
>belly fat and, 16
>brain and, 29–31
>coffee and, 86–87
>link between diet and, 7, 30
>metabolic syndrome and, 21, 30
>stress and, 33
>teas and, 88
>testosterone and, 194

amino acids:
>essential, 13, 61, 89, 152
>hGH and, 201
>proteins and, 13, 61, 89–90, 128
>supplements and, 206

andropause, 191–92

Annie's stuffed tomatoes, *168*

Annie's vegetarian wrap-for-life, *178*

antioxidants, 20, 98, 140
    coffee and, 87
    cooking and, 116–17
    melatonin and, 202
    sugars and, 67
    supplements and, 205, 208,
        213–14
    teas and, 87–88
apples, 101, 145
    BHD and, 129, 131, 133–34
    HHD and, 153, 156
    as high DIT food, 59
    juice and, 84
    Life Plan Diet shopping list
        and, 96, 99
arginine, 201, 209, 214–15
arms, 12, 15, 44–45, 46, 47
arthritis, 15, 79, 205
    essential nutrients and,
        203–4
    gluten sensitivity and, 70
    rheumatoid, 65, 203
artichokes, 96, 144
    BHD and, 131, 134–35
    HHD and, 155, 157
    JumpStart Diet and, 119, 123
Asian beans with hemp seeds,
    180
Asian cabbage salad, 175
asparagus, 37, 96, 169
    BHD and, 130, 133
    HHD and, 156–57
    JumpStart Diet and, 118,
        123
asthma, 22
atherosclerosis, 20–21, 24, 194
attentiveness, 19, 125, 136
    alcohol and, 82
    brain and, 30, 32, 34
    coffee and, 87
    teas and, 88
avocados, 64, 96, 130, 143, 154
    scallop and avocado rice bowl,
        185
    tofu and avocado rice bowl,
        185

B

bacon, 72, 106, 123
baked dishes, baked goods, 117
    baked salmon rolls, 178
    carbohydrates and, 66
    fats and, 64
bananas, 68, 100–101
Basic Health Diet (BHD), 8, 77,
    116, 125, 127–37, 140, 149,
    161–82
    Annie's stuffed tomatoes, 168
    Annie's vegetarian
        wrap-for-life, 178
    any meat meatloaf, 166
    Asian beans with hemp seeds,
        180
    Asian cabbage salad, 175
    assessing how you feel and,
        135–36
    baked salmon rolls, 178
    barbecue tuna steaks, 177
    black pepper salmon, 170
    creamy breakfast crunch, 163
    Dijon salmon, 181
    Dr. Life's Protein Pancakes,
        134, 165
    egg white omelet with fresh
        herbs, 164
    fresh mushroom salad, 166
    grilled Portobello and eggplant
        wrap, 177
    healthy greens and beans, 181
    high-powered oatmeal, 162
    lemony dill chicken breast, 169
    lentil and bean salad, 180
    Mazatlan shrimp with salsa, 167
    meals in, 127–36
    not so naked chicken, 170
    "Not So Portuguese" kale soup,
        129, 132, 168
    open-faced veggie sandwich, 167
    poached egg with smoked
        salmon, 164
    protein shakes and, 186–88
    quick salmon salad, 165

quinoa bulgur tabbouleh salad,
    171
    seitan tagine, 173
    shrimp stuffed Portobello caps,
        176
    spicy grilled summer
        vegetables, 169
    squash Italiano, 174
    steamed curried chicken, 175
    steamed curried seitan, 175
    steamed tilapia fillet, 174
    turkey stir-fry, 172
    vegan breakfast skillet, 163
    vegan chili, 179
    vegetarian stuffed peppers, 182
basil, 92, 163–64, 166, 169, 174
Baul, Ernie, 2–3
bay leaf, 184
beans, 13, 61, 69, 71
    adzuki, 94, 143, 154–55
    Asian beans with hemp seeds, 180
    BHD and, 132–34, 167–68,
        171, 178–81
    black, 94, 134, 144, 146, 155,
        167, 171, 179
    cannellini, 168, 179–81, 184
    FBD and, 143–44, 146–47,
        167–68, 171, 178–81, 184
    garbanzo, 94, 133, 147, 158, 178
    green, 96, 180
    healthy greens and beans, 181
    HHD and, 152, 154–58,
        167–68, 171, 178–81, 184
    JumpStart Diet and, 119, 123
    kidney, 94, 178–79
    lentil and bean salad, 180
    recipes and, 132–34, 143–44,
        146–47, 154–58, 167–68,
        171, 178–81, 184
    scallop and white bean gumbo,
        184
    shopping list and, 94, 96–97
    string, 97, 119, 123, 132, 146
    white, 94, 154, 157, 184
    white bean gumbo, 184
    see also soy products

exercises, exercising (*cont.*)
    of Life, 2–7, 21, 114–15, 192, 221
    metabolic syndrome and, 21
    metabolism and, 58–59
    planning tips and, 103
    proteins and, 62, 89–90
    resistance, 3, 6, 46, 59, 79, 201,
      207–8, 219
    sexuality and, 26
    stress and, 32–33
    supplements and, 205–8
    teas and, 88
    and thinking like a lean and fit
      man, 50, 53, 55
    weight loss goals and, 48–49
eyes, 18–19, 23, 65, 204, 213

F

fasting, 72–76
    eating after, 114
    5-2 diet and, 74
    JumpStart Diet and, 74–76,
      110, 113–16, 125
    of Life, 113–16, 125
    tips for, 104–5
    weight loss and, 72–74, 76,
      113–15
fat, belly, *see* belly fat
fat, body, 2, 6–8, 15, 100, 115
    aging and, 42, 44
    brain and, 30, 33
    coffee and, 87
    DEXA scan and, 46–47
    DIT foods and, 60
    exercise and, 218–19
    fad diets and, 12
    fasting and, 73–74, 114, 116
    FBD and, 77, 148
    glycemic index foods and, 68
    goals and, 8, 41, 48, 79, 148, 217
    heart disease and, 6, 42
    HHD and, 152, 159
    hormones and, 14, 16–17,
      19–20, 24, 192–95, 197–99

hunger and, 36
JumpStart Diet and, 74,
    116–17, 119, 124
and letters from Life's patients,
    78, 120, 148
of Life, 3, 42, 192, 217
measurement of, 43–45, 47
metabolism and, 57–58, 73–75
parties and, 107
percentages of, 41–42, 44–48,
    77, 110, 219
planning tips and, 102–3
proteins and, 61–62
sleep and, 23, 80
small meals and, 75–76
sugars and, 67
teas and, 88
and thinking like a lean and fit
    man, 49–50, 52
visceral, 6, 11, 44, 48
water and, 85–86
weight loss and, 43, 45, 47–48,
    50, 57, 68, 79, 102–3, 114,
    116, 148, 159, 194, 197,
    217–18
see also belly fat
Fat-Burning Diet (FBD), 8, 77,
    128, 137, 139–49, 162–88
    Annie's stuffed tomatoes, 168
    Annie's vegetarian wrap-for-
      life, 178
    any meat meatloaf, 166
    Asian beans with hemp seeds,
      180
    Asian cabbage salad, 175
    assessing how you feel and,
      147–48
    baked salmon rolls, 178
    barbecue tuna steaks, 177
    black pepper salmon, 170
    creamy breakfast crunch, 163
    Dijon salmon, 181
    Dr. Life's Protein Pancakes, 165
    egg white omelet with fresh
      herbs, 164
    exercise and, 148–49

    fresh mushroom salad, 166
    grilled Portobello and eggplant
      wrap, 177
    healthy greens and beans, 181
    herb-rubbed pork tenderloin,
      183
    high-powered oatmeal, 162
    high-protein turkey meatballs,
      183
    lemony dill chicken breast, 169
    lentil and bean salad, 180
    Mazatlan shrimp with salsa,
      167
    meals in, 141–47
    not so naked chicken, 170
    "Not So Portuguese" kale soup,
      142, 144, 146, 168
    open-faced veggie sandwich,
      167
    poached egg with smoked
      salmon, 164
    pork chops with cherries and
      almonds, 185
    protein shakes and, 141–43,
      145, 147, 186–88
    quick salmon salad, 165
    quinoa bulgur tabbouleh salad,
      171
    scallop and avocado rice bowl,
      185
    scallop and white bean gumbo,
      184
    seitan tagine, 173
    shrimp stuffed Portobello caps,
      176
    spicy grilled summer
      vegetables, 169
    squash Italiano, 174
    steamed curried chicken, 175
    steamed curried seitan, 175
    steamed tilapia fillet, 174
    turkey stir-fry, 172
    vegan breakfast skillet, 163
    vegan chili, 179
    vegetarian stuffed peppers,
      182

turkey (*cont.*)
  protein in, 61, 99
  shopping list and, 95, 99
  turkey stir-fry, *172*

U

ubiquinol, 213
United States Pharmacopeia
  (USP), 207
urine, urination, 120
  saw palmetto and, 213
  water consumption and, 86

V

vanilla:
  blueberry vanilla shake, *186*
  vanilla walnut citrus shake, *187*
vegans, 95
  HHD and, 77, 151–52, 163, 179
  vegan breakfast skillet, *163*
  vegan chili, *179*
vegetables, 63
  BHD and, 129–35, 162,
    164–69, 171–82, 187
  broth, 97, 168, 172, 179,
    181–82
  colorful, 20, 69, 124, 205, 214
  cooking of, 116
  FBD and, 141–47, 162, 164–69,
    171–84, 187
  fiber and, 71
  freezing of, 161
  glycemic indexes of, 19, 69,
    100, 161, 197
  green and green leafy, 59, 66,
    162
  healthy greens and beans, *181*
  HHD and, 152–58, 162,
    166–69, 171–84, 187
  as high DIT food, 59
  hormones and, 197, 201
  juices and, 84

JumpStart Diet and, 117–19,
    122–24
  omega-3 fatty acids and, 66
  open-faced veggie sandwich,
    167
  planning tips and, 103
  portion sizes and, 93
  recipes and, 129–34, 141–47,
    152–58, 162, 164–69,
    171–85, 187
  restaurants and, 106
  selection of, 100
  shopping list and, 92–94,
    96–100
  spicy grilled summer
    vegetables, *169*
  steamed, 106
  sugars and, 67
  supplements and, 208, 214
vegetarians:
  Annie's vegetarian wrap-for-
    life, *178*
  FBD and, 140, 178, 182
  HHD and, 151–52, 178, 182
  restaurants and, 106
  vegetarian stuffed peppers, *182*
vinaigrettes, 97, 106, 143, 153–54
vinegar:
  balsamic, 180–81
  distilled white, 97, 164
  recipes and, 134, 164, 180–81,
    185
vitamins:
  A, 83, 98, 100, 205, 209–10
  B, 82, 99–100, 205, 209
  B_1 (thiamine), 82, 201, 209
  B_2 (riboflavin), 99, 201, 209
  B_3 (niacin), 82, 99, 201, 209
  B_{12}, 152, 209
  and beverages to avoid, 82–83
  C, 98, 100, 205, 209
  D, 152, 204, 208–12
  deficiencies of, 204, 211–12
  E, 99, 205, 209–11
  as essential nutrients, 203–4,
    209

folate, folic acid, 100, 205, 209
  high dosages of, 205
  K, 209
  multivitamins, 208–14
  selection of, 207–8
  shopping lists and, 98–100,
    208–9
  supplements and, 191, 204–11
  vegans and, 152
Volkow, Nora, 37

W

waist, waistline, 1, 77, 224
  average, 44
  evaluating your current health
    status and, 26–27
  food manufacturers and, 101
  goals and, 41, 43, 48
  and letters from Life's patients,
    89, 122, 148
  measurement of, 20, 43–45,
    47–48, 120
  small meals and, 75
  teas and, 88
  see also abdomen; belly fat
waist-to-height ratio (WHtR),
    44, 47
waist-to-hip ratio (WHR), 44, 47
walking, 6–7, 27, 136, 148, 159,
    218
  fasting and, 104–5, 114–15
  hGH and, 201
  JumpStart Diet and, 124–25
walnuts, 182
  shopping list and, 95, 99
  vanilla walnut citrus shake, *187*
water, 99, 107, 128, 140, 152
  and beverages to avoid, 82
  dried fruit and, 101
  fasting and, 104–5, 113–16
  food journal and, 223–24
  Life Plan Diet goal for, 85–86,
    89
  planning tips and, 103

Live LIFE
TO THE FULLEST

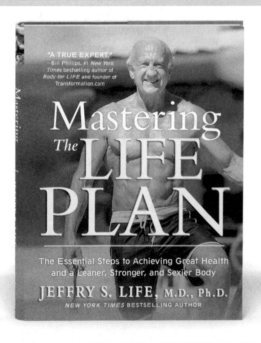

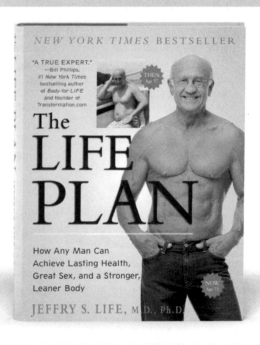